Strength To Awaken

*Make Strength Training Your Spiritual Practice
and Find New Power and Purpose in Your Life*

Robert Lundin McNamara
2nd Edition

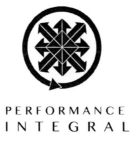

PERFORMANCE
INTEGRAL

Published by Performance Integral, Boulder, Colorado.
  www.PerformanceIntegral.com
  www.StrengthToAwaken.com

FIRST EDITION
Printed in the United States of America

2 4 6 8 10 9 7 5 3 1

COVER ART DESIGN ◆ "BRING IT DOWN"
BY
A L E X A N D R U   M U S A T
W W W . A L E X M U S A T . C O M

EDITOR-IN-CHIEF ◆ ROBERT BERG

LIBRARY OF CONGRESS CATALOGING-IN-PUBLICATION DATA

McNamara, Robert L.   1977 -
   Strength To Awaken : Make Strength Training Your Spiritual Practice and Find New
Power and Performance in Your Life / Robert McNamara

ISBN 978-0-615-54460-1

   Includes Bibliographical References (hardcover)

   1. Strength Training. 2. Human Development. 3. Performance Training.
   4. Spirituality (philosophy). 5. Psychological Development. I. Title.

Library of Congress Control Number: 2011917596

For Love.

Contents

Acknowledgements

This book has been a work in progress for about seven years. Along this path many people have supported me in countless ways; however, this work ultimately is not just a book of seven years of writing, instead it has in some ways been a culminating gesture of my practice reaching back at least two and a half decades. As such, I would like to first give thanks to the many precious individuals who have supported and challenged me throughout my life. Without the decades of turning toward daily rigorous practice, this book would never have been born.

My father first started to take me to the gym when I was in middle school. Every once in a while we would go and play racquetball and lift weights at the gym on the Ohio State University campus. My father, a campus paster at OSU in the early 1990s, would sweet-talk the student working the front desk to let me in. While I could rarely keep myself from looking backwards while playing racquetball despite my dad's instructions not to, I soaked up everything I saw and was taught in the weight room. While I had absolutely no idea at the time, my father was unexpectedly handing me what would blossom into a core spiritual discipline in my life. This is one of the most beautiful and precious gifts to receive, and I am fortunate to have received it from the man who also gave me life. Thank you, Dad.

While my father first walked me into strength training, both of my parents supported my daily engagement with physical practices. I would like to particularly thank my mother for her continued gesture of support and encouragement in my daily, year-round gymnastics training. Whether it was driving me to competitions, getting me to and from the gym every day (sometimes twice a day) or her integrative approach to excellence in both my athletics and academics, she was immensely supportive in seemingly countless ways. Without these supports, this book would not be in your hands, as much of the foundation of my explicit engagement and discipline for training was gifted to me by my first gymnastics coach, Monte Kimes. While he shaped a state champion in me during our time together, more importantly he helped birth my love and joy for embodiment and cut a groove for daily rigorous training that ultimately continues to this day.

My first athletic trainer was Ron Walter at Upper Arlington High School. Ron devoted his life to his athletes in a way that I have not seen anywhere else. Ron provided me with my first professional instruction in the methodologies of strength training. As a result, he established sound foundations from which I would build and that I carry forward in my training today. Furthermore, Ron initiated me into a tradition of continually pushing myself further in training; as a result, his contribution to my ongoing practice has been immense.

I have had many training partners over my decades of practice, and I would like to extend gratitude to all of them. They have, in their own unique ways, facilitated my training. Here are a few who played significant roles: My best friend, Chris Peraro, was the first to join me in carrying weights and a swiss ball into my first silent meditation retreat. It was here in the mountains of Colorado where we began yoking together sitting practice and strength training in an explicit fashion. In returning from retreat we fiercely explored our psychological and physiological limits in our training with a rigor I still view as pivotal in my development. My college training partner, Hunter, without who any question, was not afraid to step outside of and beyond conventions and provided a rich source of training and practice. He was also the only one on campus willing to devote as much time and energy into training as me. More recently, I would like to thank my students who began asking me for instruction in the integral discipline of strength training. Most notably I would like to thank Jamison Stone for his encouragement and Claudius Von Schroder, who has demonstrated the immense progress we are capable of when we look into the heart of strength and engage training wholeheartedly. Lastly, I would like to thank my training partner Dr. Stuart Lord for his implicit guidance in dropping all approaches in service of simply lifting.

I discovered Ken Wilber early on in college, and his work has inspired my more traditional contemplative practice outside of the weight room. His inspiring integral vision, unceasing drive for wisdom and clarity, and the integration and health of the overarching structure of life is utterly breathtaking. The opportunity to work with Ken and the Integral Institute has been life changing, life affirming and exquisitely beautiful. Ken, thanks for the passion you have sparked in my own Integral Practice and the utterly priceless contribution you are to our unfolding Kosmos.

Shawn Phillips and I met years ago as I was completing my master's degree in psychology. I was working with athletes at a number of levels and writing my thesis on the integration of developmental-constructive psychology and sport psychology. Shawn and I most readily connected on our love for strength training and a desire to liberate it from its limiting conventions. On this foundation we collaborated on a new approach to strength training that would blossom into a Gold Star Practice in the Integral Life Practice seminar series and later on in the Integral Life Practice kit. Together we placed strength training alongside many of the worlds great approaches to human transformation. Shawn, thanks for your curiosity in the further reaches of human nature and for our precious collaboration.

I would like to thank my dear friend Emily Biever who graciously supported me in taking the space to begin writing this book and who also spent thousands of hours year in and year out training with me. Additionally, Emily provided her seasoned expertise and perspective as a nutritionist, helping me to shape the direction taken on nutritional recovery. Her contributions to my practice and engagement over the years have reached beyond measure.

I would like to thank Nataraja Kallio, the head of the Yoga Department at Naropa University. Nataraja's warm friendship has been a source of rich practice in my life for over a decade now. Early on in our friendship he pointed out the deep connecting waters beneath what I do in my strength training and the great yogic tradition. His practice and yogic instruction has ushered me into the essential heart and depth of yoga, and this intersection has immeasurably contributed to the book you now hold. Thank you, Nataraja.

My dear friend and brilliant integral practitioner Cindy Lou Golin and I began collaborating on our respective writing projects, and this has been an invaluable source of support, momentum and inspiration to continue to engage the hard work of completing this book. Without her support, this book would have take much longer to complete; thank you, Cindy Lou. I would like to thank John Dupuy, who birthed the title of the book you now hold. Appropriately we had just finished our meditation practice together and were headed out to the gym later on that afternoon. My friend Sofia Diaz, who is a radiant embodiment of Integral Practice, has been a continual source of inspiration every time we connect. I would also like to thank Sofia for her rigorous practice, her sacrifice to that which reaches beyond and to the myriad ways she calls practitioners into greater embodiment. I would also like to thank Marc Gafni who has brought luminous creativity and brilliant intellectual light to my life. His philosophical teachings and probing inquiries have been a rich source of practice over the past half-decade and thus have found their way into both my training and writing.

I would like to extend my deep gratitude to Alex Musat, who has created what is perhaps the most beautiful book cover I have ever seen. Truly it is a pleasure to have my writing wrapped in this rare, precious and elegant art. Alex, thank you so much for your beautiful contribution to this book.

Rob Berg, my close friend and immensely talented editor has spent over two years working with me on refining, clarifying and structuring the book you now hold. Rob is nothing short of genius with text. The inspiring level of conceptual clarity, his understanding of writing as an art as well as his probing command for elegance in writing has touched every single word in this book. It has been a pleasure to work with his genuine Excellence, and through his work this book is able to reach into readers with much greater effectiveness and elegance. Rob, thank you. Additionally, I would like to thank Roshana Ariel for her generous editorial support in polishing this manuscript. Roshana, thank you.

My Zen teacher, Diane Musho Hamilton, has rested at the center of my heart for many years now. She is the most gifted of teachers and a beautifully immense human being. Her practice, wakefulness and rigor touches my daily practice in seemingly countless ways. Diane has profoundly and fundamentally shifted my orientation to life, experience and practice. As such this book has been implicitly shaped by her presence, instruction, love and rigor. I cannot thank her enough as the gesture of service in this book is in many ways intrinsically yoked to her service to me and her beautiful gestures of service in the world. Diane, thank you with all my heart.

My sister Deb, who has literally been there every step of my life, has been pulling and pushing upon how this text has been shaped long before I even considered writing a book. Deb's passion for life, her undying curiosity and her inspired vibrance have been a seemingly timeless guiding presence. Deb's depth of body, heart, mind and soul is nothing short of a miracle. Without her steady wisdom, I can only guess at how fundamentally lost in life I would be. Deb, thank you.

I would also like to thank my heart's great love, Brooke Gessay, who has provided me with aliveness, encouragement and beautiful support as I have completed this book. Thank you, my love.

Finally, I would like to bow deeply to my principle teacher, Death. Without the intimate confrontation with this awakening challenge I would be an empty vessel without anything of true value to share and contribute. It is with great humility that I bow in silence to your great liberation.

Rob McNamara
Winter 2011
Boulder, Colorado

Foreword

by Ken Wilber

It is a great pleasure to write this foreword. To discover strength training as an exquisitely adaptable medium of contemplation, meditation, or spiritual practice is quite extraordinary. The book you are holding in your hands redefines strength as an essential facet to the process of manifesting your greatness. It transmutes what is conventionally experienced as a mind-numbing process, focused upon largely egocentric orientations, and connects strength, true strength if you will, to the deepest awakenings of your identity and larger possibilities for yourself in life. This is the strength to awaken, and it is an absolutely beautiful way to rethink and reframe strength training.

Ultimately, genuine awakening is an arduous practice. It takes power; it takes the type of strength Rob McNamara points you toward in the following pages; it takes refocusing to find the immediateness, Presence, Being, and Mystery resting beneath the conventions that fill much of our time and effort spent in gyms and in life. Reorienting strength training as a laboratory to combine spiritual practice with performance training is a stunning realization. The book you now hold is different than virtually any type of training manual that you will pick up, particularly any book on strength training available today.

I am excited to introduce this work to you because it is a genuinely post-conventional approach to strength training, athletic performance and spiritual practice. This unconventional synthesis is precisely what makes this book so appealing and useful for readers. *Strength To Awaken* offers an entirely different attitude, awareness and philosophy to strength training. The fundamental shift in identity pointed to throughout this book fashions new perspectives for what motivates you, how you can perform at your highest levels and how you can embody excellence in the life that you are given.

What readers find in the pages that follow has in many ways been more conventionally associated with something like meditation, spirituality or contemplation. Although this book wisely and judiciously uses terms like Being, Surrender and Mystery, readers are invited to find their own sense of these terms without getting caught in the often loaded terminology associated with religious practices. As you will see, the number of opportunities to create states of *letting go* during the course of a typical strength training session is actually enormous. This book takes so many of these moments of strength training and puts them in a different perspective—of Being, of transcendence, of awakening—allowing readers to find something in what they were doing that they didn't really realize was there. McNamara's perspective is a fresh one, and strength training has yet to see a writer bring the depths of this practice to words such as in this book.

The framework provided in this book empowers readers to find that they do not need to be limited to the standard collection of benefits strength training provides, such as increased bone density, greater measures in strength and power, a more resilient immune system, an increase or preservation of muscle tissue, lower body fat percentages, along with a broad spectrum of mental and emotional benefits. While you enjoy these benefits and others, McNamara guides readers into a spiritual approach to both embodiment and performance. With new post-conventional integrated approaches such as the one you are about to explore, there is no reason you can't get both conventional and unconventional benefits at the same time.

Truly, parts of this book read more like a Rumi poem than a typical sports manual for training. Perspectives such as this are needed to allow more people to experience their larger possibilities. More than ever, we need a shift in how we approach the many moments of strength training, and this book exquisitely gives us just that; it deserves to be widely disseminated, widely read and widely used. *Strength To Awaken* is the training manual needed for awakening what the spiritual traditions generally acknowledge as the discovery of non-seeking mind. Follow the template laid out here, engage completely, and you can learn to open yourself to the infinite.

Ken Wilber
Denver, CO

Introduction

This book is about the level of qualitative engagement you can bring to your strength training and ultimately the engagement you are capable of bringing to your life as a whole. Engagement is set forth as a developmental capacity that can be refined through practice. As such, the path ahead is an exploration of how you can develop and grow as a human being through the discipline of strength training.

The trail in front of you is one characterized by a progressive deconstruction of your habituated ways of engaging your training and life. By dismantling your identification with habituation you will explore giving your body-mind's unified sacrifice to your training. This full sacrifice is one facet of engagement. Along this journey you will begin to see and inhabit the present moment with greater clarity as the clouds of habituation disperse and the vista of aliveness that is your life reveals itself to you. We are set to explore how this greater vantage point is the starting orientation for your higher levels of performance and a necessity for the level of Excellence your life already requires.

The demand of Excellence is simple: Sacrifice yourself fully into this moment. Life needs every facet of who you are, focused upon this precious moment, with complete engagement. The practice of giving all of yourself, without hesitation or reservation, is an action embodying your highest levels of maturity. Meeting this simple demand therefore requires disciplined practice. Body-Mind-Moment Training, the philosophy and system you are about to learn, is such a path of discipline and rigor.

So, what exactly is a Body-Mind-Moment and how do we train such a thing? As I will show you in the pages that follow, *you* are a Body-Mind-Moment. You are not just a body. You are not just a mind. Rather you are an integrated body-mind. As you develop your engagement to include the full unconditioned self-sacrifice of your body-mind into the present, something profound occurs. Who you are ceases to be just a limited body-mind *in* the moment. In this culminating shift you realize that you are a limited body-mind arising *as* the moment. Through this process you will have unified that which is finite with that which is infinite. This is the yoga, integration or unification of body, mind and moment as you.

This display of genuine creativity and generativity that is authentically you is trained through what we will call Integral Practice. It is through this vehicle that you will step into an integrity that faces life openheartedly, fiercely and lovingly as your strong Excellence.

As you might have guessed already, this book is not an exercise book. Conventionally understood, exercise is any activity requiring physical effort carried out with the aim of improving health and/or fitness. While strength training is unparalleled in many of its physiological measures on health and fitness, we will not be focusing upon training methodologies to slow and reverse the aging process[1], boost your basal metabolic rate[2], increase bone density[3], strengthen connective tissues and improve joint cartilage[4]. These claims among many others (such as the most worshipped: preserving and/or building muscle and accelerating fat loss) and their training strategies are available in many scientific journals, popular books and other readily available media.

We will not focus upon these conventional benefits as they are largely a distraction to the central aim in this text. We will not be entertaining ambiguous goals such as "getting in shape" or even worse, "getting in *better* shape." Nor will you find specific goals such as "losing 15 pounds," "getting a six-pack" or "increasing your one-rep max." These conventional aims bear little or no relationship to your Excellence but rather they commonly hold you firmly to the habituated means of regulating multi-layered mediocrity that is likely to govern much of your training (and life).

Exercise is largely, if not entirely, the activity of habituation that *disengages* you from precisely the discipline of engagement to be set forth in the following pages. Do not be mistaken. While this book is about strength training and you will be invited into a territory of effort you may have never conceived of, the purpose of the path ahead is not to simply improve your health, fitness or looks.

With that said, Body-Mind-Moment Training may enable you to attain conventional benefits more quickly and, yes, with less effort, but these are secondary or tertiary. I cannot stress this enough: *The coveted results that cultural lenses inscribe into their members and hoist upon pedestals are distractions.* The principle purpose for the training to be discussed can be thought of as the yoga of your Excellence. Nothing short of Excellence, which will be defined explicitly in the first chapter, suffices for this purpose. Nothing.

Your strength to awaken can be thought of as your capacity to move in congruence with your Excellence. This congruence between you and your Excellence is our chief aim together.

This is a book about serious training. The pages to follow are about the rigor, discipline and genuine joy of strength training as an Integral Practice. No facet of who you are is to be left untouched by the system you are about to learn. Physical, emotional, mental and spiritual faculties are to be enacted intentionally, refined with precision and developed through passionate wholehearted engagement.

This book is about the yoking together of your physicality with your greatest liberation. Strength training moves with spiritual practice and the integral impulse to leave no part of oneself untouched by the discipline of your heart's movement to the Divine as the Divine. This is about you transforming yourself. This is not about transforming your body as enculturated habituations often command. I steer you not into greater disloyalty to your Excellence. These words are about genuine integrative transformation. It is about you transforming yourself with intention and Surrendering to a transformation that belongs to something much greater than you likely know yourself to be. You will grow and you will be grown by something infinitely precious. This is the invitation that now reaches into you and touches your awareness.

Step into a novel emergence with me, liberate the beautiful discipline of strength training from the conventions that enslave it and millions of its practitioners who unknowingly trespass their own greatest integrity. Discover your true strength, risk everything in this pursuit, and participate in the timeless movement of embodiment awakening to that which no words can capture.

Welcome, dear friend.
Take a deep breath in and lengthen your release.
Focus your mind.
Open your body.
Settle in.

Welcome.

Part One:
Excellence: The Purpose of Life

Strength training is fundamentally not interested in getting you stronger, getting more muscle or getting in shape. To follow these common side effects, or to chase after these oft-worshipped conventional benefits is to be confused at a very basic level. Strength training is fundamentally invested not in you getting somewhere, but in you growing in your capacity to be here right now. This is the principle aim of the discipline. To miss this essential point is to miss everything. Now lift to discover the fullness of who you are right now. Train to embrace your most essential freedom.

Chapter One

The Purpose of a Human Life

If we are to look into the heart of strength training it is necessary for us to first closely examine the purpose of life. Without doing so we would likely be subjugated to the distractions of humanity as they play out within the sphere of strength training instead of exploring the essential nature of this discipline. One of our central aims here is to liberate strength training from its present distortions and fragmented habituations. To rise above the distracted life, the superficial play of human beings and the disembodied manipulation of the body, we are required to peer through these veils into the essence of our potential as human beings.

Focus through the distracted habituation of life and open your faculties of perception. Move beyond conventions and ask yourself, What is the purpose of my life? Hold this question steady in your body and mind. Do not be consumed by society's scripted answers, do not collapse into and accept your habituated comforts. To answer this perennial inquiry from these conventional faculties is to be consumed by a lesser part of you incapable of an adequate response. To answer from conventions is to answer from the dimensions of you that are categorically unable to embody the actual vitality that is your living answer. Hold this question steady, focus through the distracted human faculties and peer into the heart of you. What is the purpose of your life?

The authentic organizing purpose of life is the inhabitation of and unbounded expression of your *Excellence*. Excellence is the unique embodiment of your gifts and talents through your greatest liberation. Your greatest liberation is a freedom from the distracted habituation of the conventional ways of living. Liberation is discovered in the release of conditioning that hinders the full articulation of your gifts and talents.

We are not exploring a conventional understanding of the term excellence. The quality of being outstanding or extremely good misses the essence of what we are looking into. Nor are we are going to be consumed by the project of standing out in comparisons to others. This also in part misses the point. Excellence is not the habituated articulation of your gifts and skills done really well. While the gifts, talents and skills you have may be good and they may exceed expectations in many situations, being exceptionally good fails to stand in confidence in the face of our question at hand: What is the purpose of life?

Excellence requires your greatest liberation. It is born when you release the habituated relationship to your gifts and talents and fully embody the unique capacities that are intrinsic to you. These are not mere imitations of skillful actions you have seen others perform. These are genuine skills that are articulated only through the liberated expression of your humanity. These gifts are the expressions of your unique imprint in life. They are not your habituated attempts to outdo someone else. They are not attempts to prove yourself or establish yourself in some relative context. Your Excellence is the unique embodiment of your greatest gifts and talents that stem from the dimension of you that is fundamentally and unconditionally liberated. It is in this yoking of your greatest liberation with the articulation of your unique gifts and talents that you find the purpose of your life.

Excellence is the one overarching aim, the singular guiding principle, that calls you forth, draws you out of what you are into what you can become. Life challenges you, with each step of the way, to be more. Life never asks you to be less. Life never says: "You've shared too much"; "No thanks, your contributions aren't needed anymore"; "That's okay, you've given more than we need." Life is simply too open, incomplete and vulnerable to turn your Excellence away. In contrast, life desperately needs your Excellence. Take a look around you and I think you will see a life that is literally starving for your Excellence.

One of the great American philosophers and psychologists of our time, Abraham Maslow, once said, "If you plan on being anything less than you are capable of being, you will probably be unhappy all the days of your life."[5] Not only does the life that you live in need your Excellence, *you* fundamentally need your Excellence if you are ever to know genuine happiness, your greatest liberation and the full purpose of your life. I must warn you, if you settle for less than you are fully capable of, if you settle for the comfort of your habituations, you will be disappointed in yourself. And while I may be wrong, I doubt our world needs more disappointment in it.

Disappointment's origin often lies in conditioned patterns that divorce you from your emerging life right here and now. Habituation is the perennial obstacle to you becoming more, to you embodying your purpose in life. Intrinsic to each moment is habituation. Habituation is at its essence an automatic response. Its opposite is the conscious presence and agency for intentional action. Habituation has two sides. On the one hand, some of your automatic conditioned responsiveness is absolutely necessary for your fluid functioning in life. On the other hand, some of the automated responses deteriorate your conscious presence and erode your capacity to intentionally direct your life. As we explore habituation, we will be largely focused upon the latter negative function of your conditioned responses.

Some form of conditioned way of being, acting and negotiating life is always arising. These habituations are, however, not the entirety of you. Yes, they are a part of you, however we all too often mistake these routine parts of ourselves for the whole, and when this fallacy is made, inevitably the unbounded vitality that is your greater life erodes into a dim habituated vitality that is often in direct conflict with your Excellence.

As habituation is an intrinsic part of the human condition, we find a poignant necessity for something to unknot our identification with our conditioned patterns, stories and preferences that dominate so much of the conventional lives we lead. Something is required to draw you from empty habit to the full and liberated vitality of your Excellence. This something is *Strength*.

Strength: Your Vehicle Toward Excellence

Strength is, at its core, animated through two mediums: Doing and Being. We often think of strength as being able to physically perform some extraordinary feat, or we see strength through an emotional lens when we see someone who is able to weather the high storms of life with grace and skill. Other times we recognize strength as the capacity to harness the focus, will, and determination to persevere amidst daunting obstacles. While these are all expressions of strength (they beautifully highlight physical, emotional, and mental dimensions of strength), they all focus upon Doing and leave out Being. Strength's essential ground, and the foundation of every expression of genuine strength, is rooted in Being. Strength's most profound expression, and its most simple expression, is in the capacity to Be.

Let us talk about you for a moment. You are sitting reading this book. You may be at home in your favorite chair reading under the soft light radiating from the lamp shade. You might be reading in a coffee shop amidst the subtle buzz of energy with people talking, sipping their favorite beverages, catching up on the latest news, or any number of alternative ways of reading these words. You are right where you are.

There is a certain obviousness to this; you cannot be anywhere else if you are right here, correct? On a physical level, you being here is pretty obvious, simple, and unavoidable. While this is part of the picture, this is not the fundamental ground of strength. When we start to investigate the other layers of who you are, things get a little more complicated. Let us hypothetically say you have gone through a breakup, and you have left your heart, passion, and love with someone else. Emotionally, you may not be fully here as you read these words. Maybe you are drained, depleted, and exhausted from a move, or some other major transition. Again, if this is the case, you may not be fully present as you read this book.

Let us look at another layer of you: your mind. Let us say you are really excited about a new project at work, a new relationship, or perhaps the birth of a child. As you read these words your mind drifts off planning how you are going to proceed with your day. Or, maybe work is particularly stressful, and you are chewing on how to approach a difficult situation with a boss or someone who reports to you. As your eyes flow across these words, your mind focuses upon the unfolding dilemma and works on a potential solution. Again, your body is here, but your mind is not fully here if some event is pulling attention away from these words.

Emotionally and mentally *being* here is a little bit more complicated. As you are able to divorce yourself from this moment in anticipation of what is to come, or to attempt to make sense of something that has happened in the past, you are not fully here. Right now, in this moment, rate yourself. How present are you emotionally? How present are you mentally? Give yourself a number, 1 representing you as completely somewhere else, 10 representing you as fully present and engaged.

When you stop being present emotionally and/or mentally, you lose part of your strength. You lose your fundamental capacity to relate to, and be with, what is happening right here and right now. When you are emotionally or mentally disconnected from the present moment, your ability to be here is compromised and thus strength washes away, leaving a ghostly phantom behind. The guiding orientation is your habitual conditioning. You are on autopilot. Physically you may "be" present, but a significant chunk of you is largely missing-in-action. Your quality of life suffers, your ability to perform at high levels is stunted, and your precious life, vibrating within and about you, slips by largely unnoticed.

While your emotional and mental capacity to "be" here is centrally important, we have yet to discuss the fundamental ground of strength. Beyond the thinking mind, beyond your emotional conditioning is a territory of Being itself. This limitless field of presence is your capacity to both witness and inhabit what is. This is, at the core, one of your most essential assets. This is especially the case when we consider what can liberate you from the habituation of your body, mind and life.

If you are to know your Excellence, you must be willing to cultivate the full spectrum of your strength. You require the full resources available to you if you are to consistently move through the veil of habituation to refine your articulation of Excellence. To do so is to answer one of life's central calls for you to awaken to something more than you are right now. In doing so, you will move into the unbounded territory of yourself and life that embodies your Excellence.

Chapter Two
The Storm & Your Awakening

It is late October. The leaves on the trees have turned color and have begun to fall to the ground. I am a seventh-grader tenuously walking into a new school. My family and I have just moved east from central Illinois to a suburb of Columbus, Ohio. School had never been much of a social place for me as all of my close friendships in Illinois were born through gymnastics, not school. Here I was opening the front door to Hastings Middle School wondering, "Who is going to be my friend?" and "Am I going to fit in here?"

Within this transition from known to unknown, something significant began to unfold. It was here in Upper Arlington Ohio that I started to wake up. By day, in my awkwardness of finding ways to fit in to a new school, I started to peer into what I valued. By night, as I drifted off to sleep alone in my basement bedroom, another journey, this one much more profound, was unfolding.

From the emptiness of sleep, my body jolts upward as I gasp for air. Like a knife cutting through space, my awareness sharply slices into my waking life, and with a seamless movement I roll forward to the foot of my bed tumbling out onto the floor.

The storm is here.

I feel as though I am only breathing in and out of my mouth, unable to breathe air into my lungs. I crawl across the floor carefully to conserve energy, yet swiftly to preserve precious time. My lungs feel locked shut. I reach the white bookcase built into my bedroom wall, grab my nebulizer, insert the mouthpiece, and turn on the only thing that can save me in this moment. Medicine vapor pours out of the mouthpiece, and I stare eye to eye into the storm. There is nowhere to go, no way to avoid, and no place to hide. I begin inhaling, and it is excruciating, a burning in my chest like nothing I have ever experienced.

Nothing else exists right now in the immediacy of this crisis. I hunch over my legs, left hand resting on the floor, fingers digging into the carpet. My shoulders rise and back muscles clench like rocks to help me breathe. My neck tenses as I exert all my effort in taking air and medicine into my lungs. My in-breath feels empty, the pain intensifies and a tremendous heat flashes through my body.

Something holds me to a calm focus.

As I exhale the small amount of air in my lungs, I feel a slice of eternity. Time slows as the pain dissipates to the background. Breathing out is effortless, and in these few brief moments I know stillness and peace. In the center of the storm, for a brief moment, I am okay.

At the transitional space from the bottom of my out-breath to the top of my in-breath the center of the storm shifts away and I once again am consumed in turbulence. I desire to let go, to give up rather than brave the winds of this pain, yet I have little choice in the matter now. I am forced into another in-breath.

My shoulders rise and expand, I clench my back and rock forward, my legs folded underneath me. I draw in whatever air I am able to get as the burning struggle returns and intensifies. My eyes fill with tears and I cry without sound. Cold sweat covers my body as I fight and claw for each breath. Each out-breath brings with it a cool, relaxing break from the pain and intensity. The suffocation, agony and stabbing constriction drifts into the background of my experience waiting to surface again. Moments pass as if years.

In time the storm begins to dissipate. My breathing starts to become natural and I notice an intrinsic joy as each breath slowly and easily rises and falls. The storm has passed; however, I intuit this is not my last encounter. Something in me knows I will dance with death again.

Asthma was my call for awakening. I had attacks for years before these calls to contemplate my life and death would be answered with any serious consideration, but it was in the seventh grade that I finally awoke to a basic human condition: I am going to die. And for me, as I walked through the awkwardness of middle school, I thought to myself, "Tonight might be my time."

This fact of life is an essential part of the felt sense of *being* alive. Part of the difference among us is that we feel and know this truth to different degrees and in different ways. Ultimately, we all have our own individual paths to death; it is just that some of us are further along than others. And while we often look at those facing death with some form of pity, it is really those who avoid death the most that suffer the greatest losses in life.

Death offers an appreciation, grace and confidence that simply cannot be matched by anything else. There is no substitute or shortcut.

My encounters with death through the vehicle of asthma have been among my greatest teachers. Through these formative experiences and countless hours of contemplation, I began cultivating a clarity about life, how I needed to live it, and what really mattered to me. As many of my friends in middle school talked about rumors, designer sneakers, and Friday night parties, I was asking myself, "Am I going to be alive tomorrow?" and, "If so, what is most important for me right now?"

Asthma attacks most often happened in the middle of the night, when my adrenaline levels would naturally drop and sleep allowed me to overlook important signs such as the subtle deterioration in the quality of my breathing. I would not awaken until I was well into a crisis.

I started asking myself, "What if the next time I wake up too late?" "If this was my last day, did I live it well?" "Did I spend it in a way that made it truly worthwhile?" Once I started to respect, honor and explore my calls to awaken, the stability of my mind began to grow, and along with it, clear answers to many of the core questions life presented me.

I lived my life one day at a time, and one of the central commitments to myself was that if this was indeed my last day I might as well spend it being happy. This approach empowered me to take responsibility for how I felt. I knew I could not just do whatever I wanted, but I did have the clarity that I could choose to be happy regardless of what situation I found myself in.

As I confronted the possibility of not waking up the next morning, I found myself experiencing a fuller life. I lived with greater intentionality and consideration of how to conduct myself, how to step a little more fully into my life and how to enjoy each day.

We all have calls to awaken, confront and engage ourselves and our lives more fully. It may be the death of a loved one, or perhaps a car accident you survived, or a life-threatening condition. You may have suddenly found your heart open to the sight of an animal dying, losing a job that you have poured all of yourself into, or seeing an intimate relationship end. Regardless of what form your call takes, you have probably had one, if not many, invitations to open your eyes and awaken to a territory beyond habituation.

When you start to answer these calls, you may begin to see that your answers depend upon a mixture of choice and grace, intention and inspiration, ability and necessity. As you begin to explore the central purpose of your life with greater depth, you need to connect to your own living pulse. You simply must feel your call to live your purpose more fully as an intrinsic necessity, and nothing impels the urgency of your Excellence with more power than the unmediated confrontation with death. You must find how death is calling you to sacrifice who you are for the greater Excellence that you can participate with right now.

Without a connection to the urgent necessity that death creates, you will often find yourself with only half of the equation necessary to cut through the habituation and step into your Excellence. Without awakening to your deeper calling, you will have choice without grace, intention without inspiration, ability without necessity. One without the other is not going to birth the Excellence your heart yearns for and that holds the capacity to transform your training, catalyze higher performance capacities and/or create a new level of happiness, authenticity and realization.

So, ask yourself: What is my call to awaken more fully to life?

Are you ready to engage and articulate your life's purpose more fully? Are you ready to take bold action? Are you ready to sacrifice who you are right now for the chance to manifest something much more precious and elegant? Or are you going to allow your Excellence to atrophy as your habituated existence washes life, vibrance and vitality away?

If you are ready to cut through to your emerging Excellence, let us begin by examining some of the central habituations that fracture Excellence from your embodiment moment to moment. By examining some of the fundamental strategies that habituation uses to collapse your vitality and potential, we will begin to open the door to the greater possibilities of strength training and your budding Excellence.

Chapter Three

The Myth of Disengagement & The Lie of Happiness

Your ego, or your conventional belief systems, habitual thought patterns and traditional way of being in the world, creates the myth of disengagement, as well as the lie of happiness. These pervasive deceptions are habituations that cannot be clearly seen by your ego. Just as a camera cannot take a picture of itself, the ego cannot see this illusion because the activity of ego *creates* this illusion. The illusion of disengagement is part of the ego's embedded unconscious[6], it is a byproduct of the most basic processes of your ego, which at the core is a struggle with the present moment. Moment to moment the ego creates an imagined future or an imagined past that is fundamentally different from the situation you are actually in right now. As such your ego is a repository for the habituated ways of functioning that often cut the live connection to your Excellence.

While more and more people are having temporary experiences that glimpse beyond their ego's conditioning, most people have yet to shift their everyday functioning beyond the conventional stages in which the ego's struggle is the dominant volitional center of gravity. Consequently, when you look around, you see the pervasiveness of the myth of disengagement being played out.

The myth of disengagement often manifests as an imagined or projected future in which happiness results from the disengagement from life, responsibilities and everyday routines. This is the ego's lie of happiness. Unfortunately your undying desire for happiness will never be satisfied as long as life is dictated by the lens of your ego's habituation. The truth is authentic happiness and your larger purpose as a human being are rarely in alignment with what is most comfortable for your ego. And comfort, not happiness, is what your habituation actually seeks. As a result, the Excellence you and your life need and desire will not stem from egoic activity.

At a basic level, ego continually sets up an adversarial relationship to the present moment. This basic struggle with what is happening right here and now will manifest in more and more subtle and sophisticated ways as you grow and develop.

Vacations are one example of this pervasive myth and illusion in which the belief of abandoning your everyday existence will lead to happiness. The conventional sense of self believes changing your surroundings is going to automatically change your interior experience. That is, of course, if the place has the amenities and experiences you are expecting. While this may work for a short while, it does not take long to encounter the sobering realization that you have carried all the baggage you wanted to leave at home and at the office with you. Not to mention you have not taken a vacation from the struggle your ego generates with family or your partner, if you happened to bring them along. They are not the root cause of your struggles anyway. The root of the problem lies within you. Struggle is the ground, the foundation, of your habituated and conventional sense of self. As you will see, it is this foundation that is incapable of true happiness.

So, why does your ego struggle?

The ego has no choice but to act out the processes that constitute its identity and function. The entire conventional self is built upon a plethora of tensions among various polarities. A conventional self can rattle off thousands of these tension points at a moment's notice:

I like the warm sun and hate the cold.
I love spicy food and hate steak and potatoes.
I like quality products with style and despise Walmart.
I like Earth-friendly products and do not want anything with chemicals in it.
I like cheap airline tickets and hate paying an arm and a leg to see family over the holidays.
I like short lines and hate waiting.
I like big meals and hate being hungry.
I like being wealthy and hate being poor.
I love coffee in the morning and hate when I do not get it.

"I like this; I dislike that." As long as your sense of self and identity remains tied to the ego, you are largely going to be locked into this perpetual stance of struggle. Can you hear and feel your own habituated sense of self and how you create your egoic identity through this constant play of preferences?

Returning to our vacation example, it is only a matter of time before your rejection of, struggle with and aversion to the immediate present moment starts to reject the vacation more and more. Things go wrong, expectations are not met and swiftly the habitual thought patterns of a well-seasoned ego will introduce the "What if ..." wave of attacks:

What if this was different?
What if this did or didn't happen?
What if that person just would have acted differently?
Perhaps then you will be or would have been happy.

The conventional self has a particularly strong habituated tendency to project happiness into just about anything that does not exist in this moment, even in the most beautiful of settings. Sadly, amidst this sea of struggles, your life passes by. As each moment passes, a beautifully rich and unique opportunity for true happiness slips by unrecognized. The ego lies to you about where happiness presumably resides as your conditioning wrestles with acquiring this and eliminating that.

Another domain in this struggle is retirement. The ego will sacrifice just about anything and everything to attain its perceived fantasy, a life devoid of responsibility. Consequently the ego will struggle hard for years in hopes of finally attaining the retirement of its dreams (or what the ego is hoping true happiness to be).

For many people, retirement represents the freedom the ego pretends to desire yet unconsciously fears more than anything. Freedom is desired by the ego because it is something that it can always project happiness into. The ego will conflate happiness and freedom because your ego will never possess freedom. Freedom resides only in the immediacy of each and every moment, and this immediacy is one of the core fears the ego possesses. Thus, with regard to happiness, egoic habituation avoids precisely what it seeks.

However, if you strengthen and reinforce the ego, do not expect anything but superficial changes. Changes in jobs, changes in relationships, moving to a new part of the world, retiring, going on vacation, etc., do not shift your relationship with the ego's fundamental position in the world in an enduring way. What happens when you achieve these ends? You may have a transient experience of satisfaction, but ultimately these external changes fail to relieve you of the conditioned struggle, and so now happiness resides somewhere else and the habituation continues.

Take a look at the ego's way of functioning in intimate relationships. Instead of enjoying the human being who has chosen to be with you, the habituated struggle of your ego wants them to be sexier, more successful in the world, more emotionally responsive, less critical, and so on. "If they were more of this and less of that, then I'd be happy with them." Maybe you did not find what you were looking for and so you leave and choose a new partner only to find out that this road leads you to the same familiar territory. Maybe you got married and have a family and just keep on pressing repeat, desiring for your partner to be different in some way. Or perhaps the ego's struggle has become critical of yourself in relationship. "If I could only get rid of this part of myself, then I'd be happy," or, "If I could improve this part, then I'd probably be happy in my relationship."

Regardless of whether you look into your vocation, relationships or life as a whole, following your ego's habituated commitment to struggle severs you from both your happiness and Excellence. Your greatest achievements, your highest levels of performance, the most elegant expressions of your beauty and confidence, the most skillful negotiation of life are not born through your unconscious, conditioned and unending struggle. Struggling to disengage from what is actually here rarely generates the genuine Excellence your life is calling for and the happiness your heart is sincerely drawn to. No amount of habituated struggle can give birth to the Excellence your heart seeks within.

Excellence is calling you to qualitatively show up with greater strength. Strength is the vehicle through which you can pierce the perennial obstacle of your habituation propelling you into the greater aliveness of your Excellence. Strength, an intrinsic dimension of Excellence, is animated through the active conscious *engagement* of your unique gifts and skills. Refining your capacity to effectively and efficiently act upon your purpose is central to your Excellence. Equally important is strength's essential foundation: your capacity to Be. Being is, at its center, your greatest liberation. Your true strength is an invitation to participate with the happiness that resides right here in this moment beyond your conditioned struggles. Strength and Excellence move in concert; they mutually depend upon one another and mutually reinforce each other. It is here that we begin to see the seeds of the essential nature of the rich discipline of strength training and the path into your emerging Excellence.

Chapter Four

True Happiness

True happiness is not the same thing as the superficial fleeting experiences of happiness. Nor is it projects of maintaining comfort, for the heart of happiness can be said to be the complete opposite of comfort.

True happiness is the complete acceptance of, and engagement with, the present moment. As such the ego's habituated struggle is fundamentally at odds with your true happiness. To realize this is to dramatically clarify your life.

The ego has varying degrees of distortion and connection with the present moment. There are times when your habituated egoic struggle is less overt and retains a more subtle conflicted stance toward the arising present moment. In these times you may have a fairly accurate view of the world around you and you may have a relative experience of happiness. However, if someone triggers your ego with some challenging feedback, your connection with what is really happening can rapidly disintegrate, and along with it your ego's fragile experience of contentment. When this happens, the ability to relate to what is really happening quickly erodes into a distorted view of reality. Generally speaking, the more triggered the ego is, the more distorted and warped your view becomes and the less contact you have with the originating source of happiness.

When the ego is "triggered" some event has accentuated the ego's conflicted and defensive stance toward the present moment. Typically the ego focuses exclusively on this charged stimulus and abandons any other possible perspectives. The orientation your ego will tend to adopt toward this person, system or event is as a personal attack, triggering a felt need to protect and defend itself.

Instead of being attuned to the full field of what is arising, you only consciously relate to a small portion of what is happening and unconsciously allow your habituation to govern your life.

There is a range, or spectrum, of the ego's degree of connection to the present moment. On one end you have a non-triggered state in which the ego retains a fairly adequate view of the conventional world around you. While the ego never has an intimate relationship with what is actually occurring (because the basic ground of ego's struggle distorts what is present in the moment), you are able to create a generally functional perspective. Somewhere in the middle of this continuum the ego becomes agitated. The shift from a mild agitation to a triggered state accentuates the narrowing of attention and the heightening of a struggle with various dimensions of experience. In the triggered state a largely unconscious response from the ego's conditioning takes control thus determining the course of your decisions and actions. On the other end of this spectrum we find a highly triggered state in which the ego almost completely closes down and dissociates from the present moment. As the blind unfolding of your conditioning drives all the decisions in your life you unknowingly follow the ego's most base attempts to regain safety and security. What ends up playing out are habitual defense tactics, often the ones you learned in the first few years of life, only now your ego has been repeating them for decades, regardless of the degree of their effectiveness in life.

The more your ego's attention narrows and closes, the less contact it has with what is actually happening and the more habituated your response. Ultimately the more triggered the ego becomes, the less you are able to attune to the full territory of yourself and your life.

The central point here is that the ego never has a completely attuned view of the present moment because of its fundamental struggle, continually introducing distortion, and thus the ego is fundamentally unable to know true happiness. The complete acceptance of and engagement with the truth of your direct experience slips by.

The fact of the matter is this: You must function beyond ego if you are to know the heart of genuine happiness. Many of us can relate to these precious moments. Even if these suspensions of our egoic struggle last only a brief second, they often leave lifelong memories. Whether these moments are those first steps down the aisle as you look toward your soon-to-be husband, an effortless shot right at the buzzer that wins the game, watching your child take her first step or, if you are like me, feeling the open bliss of doing a pull-up, the center of happiness remains the same in its ability to cut through your habituation.

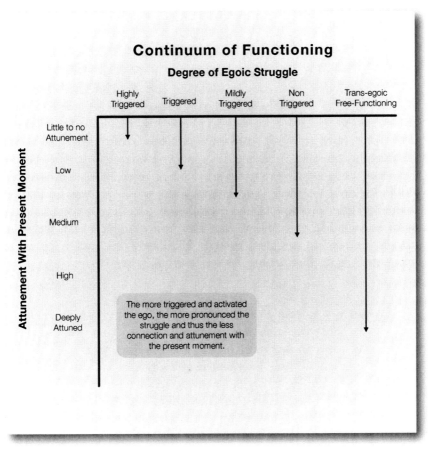

When your awareness disidentifies from your conditioned functioning, you have states, or transitory experiences, where you metabolize life more fully. In these moments you can enjoy a level of happiness and bliss that is not dependent upon any action, a level of happiness the ego is fundamentally unable to know intimately yet will endlessly pursue like a dog chasing its tail.

These glimpses beyond the conditioned self are not necessarily the result of doing something. It is not the result of disengaging from your day-to-day life nor is it the result of accomplishing some great feat or removing some heavy obligation. Knowing yourself beyond your habituated conditioning is often born through your engagement with your life through the inhabitation of Being. It is through Being's unconditioned presence that you come to know, feel and embody true happiness. Radiant joy and unbounded happiness stem from the engaged embodied presence of Being.

While you can wait around for the occasional glimpse into your larger potential, it could be years before you are genuinely happy again. For example, if you established a perspective with yourself that you were never good enough in grade school because of some pivotal feedback from a parent, teacher or coach, you might end up being an overachiever in many areas of your life. In high school you strived diligently to make honors and to get into a top-notch college. Athletically you trained and performed hard to gain recognition from scouts and to obtain scholarships. In college you might double-major to again compensate for feeling as though you were not good enough. After college you get your foot in the door to a promising company and work your way up through promotion after promotion, and even though you have accomplished so much in your life, you still, at your core, are struggling with feeling as though you are just not good enough. Ultimately this reinforcing of the habituated egoic functioning makes your glimpses beyond ego much more difficult.

An alternative is to take your conditioned history head-on, to challenge yourself to face your habitual thought patterns, your limiting belief systems and conventional sense of self that reinforce your ego's struggle with this moment. If this intention is to be picked up and carried out regularly and wholeheartedly, an alternative stance can be discovered, cultivated and refined. Your body and mind can find a stance that is more effective, efficient, rewarding and enjoyable, one that connects you intimately with the unbounded happiness of the center of your Being.

Along the way you will come to intimately know the difficulty of learning how to shift the most basic stance toward yourself, your life and those with whom you share this precious gift. In the process, you will learn how to live in, act from and perform with the presence of Being fueling your greatness. True happiness could stop being a special occasion and instead be the everyday reality that radiates from your Excellence.

This alternative is a viable option for you, though it is not easy. But it is a joyous and purposeful one. The intention to cultivate this new stance that transcends the conventional self is within the heart of your Excellence and at the center of your purpose in life. With this sole intention, life can take on entirely new dimensions. It is within these novel dimensions that you will uncover and give birth to your ever-refining Excellence.

And odd as it may seem, in the process of liberating yourself from habituation, you will attain the skills and capacities to acquire the objects of your ego's desires much more swiftly and with greater ease. Without the constant struggle embedded within the ego's functioning driving your life, you will experience progress the ego cannot even fathom. While the conventional sense of self is most likely excited by this prospect, as you mature you will come to understand the dual nature of these accomplishments. These "steps forward" trigger the conventional sense of self and ultimately force you to further refine yourself and your training. Before this refinement happens, you are likely to get stuck, and while there is no bad place to get stuck along the journey beyond your ego, there are no good places to get stuck either.

Regardless, the sole intention to cultivate a new relationship with the present moment holds a key to the joyful embodiment of the purpose of your life. While this intention carves forth a new possibility for you, something else is required for you to answer the call of Excellence.

Chapter Five
The Necessity of Practice

Practice is preparation. Without practice the human being is unprepared to meet the demands of life. While some species are born "hard-wired" to operate maturely as soon as they enter life, human beings require practice. Nature provides a crocodile with all the necessary capacities to survive as soon as they are born. For all practical purposes a newborn crocodile is an adult crocodile, just smaller. In contrast, human beings require complex exchanges between nature and nurture over decades of experience to cultivate mature capacities. Of the full territory of being human, the majority of life is intrinsically tied to skills that are learned and refined through repeated practice over a diverse range of faculties.

Practice is, at its center, *engagement*. When you practice you engage the various faculties that the chosen activity requires. The more you engage, the more prepared you become. When you took your first steps in life and began walking, you most likely balanced tentatively, teetered and fell. Often. But with practice, as you engaged the activity of walking over and over, you became increasingly more competent, more proficient and ultimately more elegant to move about in the world and meet the demands of your life.

So what happens if you do not practice? Without practice you often find yourself lacking the competence needed to meet the multifaceted challenges of life. Fail to engage your sexuality and most likely your partner will soon ask for more than you are prepared to offer. Fail to engage in disciplining your mental focus and you are likely to find yourself putting out distracting fires at work instead of focusing on real strategic priorities. Fail to practice attuning to your child and you are likely to find yourself unprepared in being able to connect with them as they grow.

Without the repeated engagement of practice you are largely unprepared to meet the demands of your life. It is simple; practice is a necessity. But what happens when you engage life and acquire a certain level of competency that is satisfactory for you? To answer this question we must look more closely into what it means to engage.

Engagement is the conscious inhabitation of your body and mind. Practice is happening when your open awareness is moving with, in and through your embodied activity. Intrinsic to practice is your conscious participation with your life. Engagement is the conduction of your free and open awareness through your activities, whatever they may be.

When you acquire a certain level of competence that is presumed to be satisfactory, practice typically stops. As soon as "good enough" is achieved something subtle yet extremely powerful happens: Habituation steps in. One of your habituation's central attachments is comfort. Wherever you are comfortable, wherever "good enough" is subjectively perceived, your habituation will invest vast amounts of resources to maintain this comfortable status quo. One way your ego achieves this is to stop practicing.

Suddenly, the practice that birthed the greater competence in your life stops and your conditioning steps in. As engagement ceases, the conscious participation and inhabitation of your body, mind and life is replaced by your ego's habituation. And as soon as you cease consciously metabolizing your experience within the direct immediacy of the present moment, you are no longer preparing yourself—your ego is just *repeating* itself.

Life's vivid textures, the alive energy and unbounded beauty, fade. The result is that hours pass, then weeks and entire months float by, years and sometimes entire decades pass, with the same patterns repeating. One song is on repeat seemingly playing without end. You are not becoming more prepared through greater refinement but rather more prepared to execute the same habituated pattern regardless of what demands are present.

So while practice is a necessity for survival, it is often only a matter of time before your ego steps in and habituation hijacks your engagement with life. Fortunately, given the trap of your ego's investment in comfort, there is a second dimension to answering this question.

The second reason we practice is because of a desire, a seeking to improve, a yearning to refine and develop ourselves and the world we live in. Survival is not enough for human beings. There is some facet of humanity that is intrinsically invested in creativity. The human drive for progress is interested in fashioning some dimension of oneself and life anew, taking what is not here and merely a possibility and making it an actuality.

If you look closely, cutting through your ego's habituated attempts to struggle with this dimension of yourself and that dimension of life, I think you will find a simple impulse, drive or inner imposition that lives within your heart. This force is an energy that continually draws you forward, inspires you out of the limitations and constraints present and into a greater, more liberated, fullness of life. This impulse is congruent with the present moment; it is not in conflict as the ego's position maintains. Instead of struggle, this force moves through uninhibited participation with the truth of your direct experience. This inspired force moves with that which is good, true and beautiful. This dimension of you is perhaps the central reason that you practice even when you have developed adequate skills to function with grace and efficiency in society.

This inspired desire to refine yourself, the inner imposition to develop and evolve your gifts, skills and unique capacities, is nothing other than your Excellence calling you forth into your greatest articulations. Your desire to go beyond habituation, to reach into novelty and to liberate the constraints of your life is the beating heart of your true strength. When you free yourself from the ego's grip on comfort, I think you will find yourself realizing a necessity once again. If you are to actually face and embody the purpose of your life, you need your strength. Without practice, strength and Excellence rarely manifest. Ultimately, practice is part necessity and part inspiration. To understand and embody practice requires both.

Integral Practice

While practice cultivates greater preparation and engagement resulting in the refinement and development of yourself, the skills you possess and the capacities you can enact in your life, there is a catch. You refine only the dimensions of yourself that you are engaging in practice. So while you may be incredibly focused on one area of your life, another equally important dimension may be stuck in habituation. While this may result in a high degree of competence in one area, if central dimensions of you are not refined through practice, inevitably you will find yourself lacking essential competencies for addressing the true demands of the full scope of your life.

Integral Practice is a technology that addresses these inherent limitations of practice by engaging all of the major dimensions of yourself. By engaging all of these facets, you will be able to unfold, develop, refine and actualize your larger potential with greater efficiency.

One of the ways Integral Practice has been utilized is through the lens of cross training in athletics. Serious athletes are dogged about performance, and as such they are grounded in objective measurements. What athletes discovered was that every approach to training has both strengths and weaknesses. To train in just one approach left dimensions of their athletic capacity untrained. When their sport demanded responses from them that their training methodology did not address adequately they found themselves unprepared.

For example, marathon runners who train only long runs and do not develop their ability to sprint explosively for shorter durations have at least one glaring weakness. If the race comes down to sprinting speed during the last 200 meters to the finish line, the athletes who failed to cultivate their capacity to sprint will find themselves unprepared and outperformed. This is especially the case if their competition had been training both capacities.

Cross training has become an embedded dimension to athletics because of its positive impact upon recovery from training[7], its application with injury prevention[8] as well as its ability to optimize performance[9,10]. Athletes at most levels now employ some form of cross training for a more integrated approach to meeting the full demands of their sport. As a result athletes enjoy competing at entirely new levels. By training what may at first appear to be seemingly unrelated dimensions of themselves, they enjoy novel performance capacities when it is time to compete.

For example, some National Football League players cross train with dance and ballet to improve athleticism on the field. One effective form of cross training for soccer involves martial arts. There are National Hockey League teams who cross train their professional athletes with yoga in addition to their on-ice training. Strength training is one dimension of cross training that many sports employ today to improve performance.

While cross training typically focuses exclusively on training physical capacities, Integral Practice looks to engage all of the major human faculties, not just the physical. Integral Practice spans across the physical, emotional, relational, mental and spiritual dimensions of selfhood. There are two ways to look at and enact Integral Practice, and both are absolutely essential to this discipline. The first, and perhaps the most widely understood, is that Integral Practice is the *sequential* engagement of all of your major faculties. This means that each of the major dimensions of yourself are regularly practiced separately.

You may begin by practicing with your physical capacities, pouring your open consciousness into your kinesthetic skills and movement capacities. Developing your strength, endurance, balance or flexibility are all different dimensions of kinesthetic skills you may cultivate. Later on you choose to engage your emotional faculties with the intention to develop your emotional intelligence. This may involve increasing your ability for emotional self-control, improving your ability to generate initiative and positive motivation in your life or refining your capacity to be adaptive in the face of stress. Next, your relational or interpersonal faculties could be developed by expanding your capacity for empathy, clear precise communication or improving your ability to manage conflict in relationship. Mental faculties may later on be engaged and refined through rigorous intellectual study and investigation. Through this process you step outside of your own perspective thus expanding your ability for perspective-taking. You may decide to refine your ability for strategic thinking as you develop plans to execute in your career or enhance your ability to perceive and understand complexity as you investigate the work of experts in your field. Finally, you may close your day in contemplation or meditation as you develop your spiritual faculties. You may rigorously focus your mind into a singular intention as you refine your faculties of perception to penetrate into the essence of life or you may center your attention and presence into the inner room to dwell in God's presence as you practice centering prayer.

In this way your central faculties are regularly strengthened. This daily practice breathes more life into your body and mind, balances and integrates your development[11], and accelerates the rate at which you can shift your life to the next level[12]. Ultimately Integral Practice is a powerful vehicle for bringing your fullest, most free expression of your unique gifts, talents and skills into the world. Fail to pursue an Integral Practice and you will likely leave important dimensions of yourself undeveloped or underdeveloped. If you look into the most painful parts of your life, the areas where you struggle the most, you will often find some central faculty or set of faculties that are not developed enough to adequately respond. Simply put, a lack of practice almost always leads to pain in some area of your life.

The second way to look at and enact Integral Practice is the more important perspective to understand if you are to answer the true call for Excellence with graceful efficiency and effectiveness. Integral Practice understood and lived from the sequential perspective is important, yet the heart of Integral Practice is something else. The essential aliveness of Integral Practice resides in the engagement of all of your major faculties in the *immediacy* of the moment and your present activity.

Through this understanding, you can inhabit the true elegance of Integral Practice. Regardless of what you are doing, you have the capacity to practice with the full territory of your Being. Whether you are running, at work in front of your computer, making love, in a board meeting or playing with your children, your embodiment is accessible for your full participation. Your relational faculties can be engaged through connecting with the direct truth of your immediate experience. Similarly, your mental and emotional faculties are always available for your conscious engagement and full participation. Finally, your spiritual essence, the seat of your most open and liberated consciousness, is an essential fabric of what it means to genuinely practice in an integrative way.

Integral Practice from this perspective has no end, only a beginning ... followed by another beginning. This path requires a constant unwavering commitment to engage. While this may appear tiresome, I can assure you, this is the only path from which you will truly and fully understand rest, and the complete release of Surrender, the letting go of the ego's compulsive struggle. Sadly, the alternative is the continued unconscious investment in your ego's unwavering habituated struggle with the truth of what is and the deception that this process of grappling can eventually result in genuine happiness.

This book is about the tool of strength training birthed as an Integral Practice and how this path can foster your emergent Excellence. In the process we will liberate strength training from the habituated conventions that currently trap this discipline and millions of its practitioners. Whether you are an elite athlete, someone struggling to find your motivation to "get in shape," a busy executive who has discovered you live your life "disembodied," or a seasoned strength trainer burnt out on an old paradigm, this book has something important for you and your ever-emergent Excellence. Even if you have never even considered strength training as a viable option for your life (if you prefer yoga or meditation, as examples), this book has something priceless to offer.

If you are to know the full unbounded truth of your Excellence, the path outlined in the pages to follow illustrate how you can step into your own unique embodiment of strength training as an Integral Practice. As a result you will learn how to bring your integrated engagement to the full territory of your life. You will discover how to Surrender your habituation and your conventional ways of functioning through ego for the larger field of life and Being that is calling out to you.

Part Two:
Transforming Your Training

As I draw air into my lungs, my ribs expand.
My spine arches opening my heart toward
the earth. I stop. As I hold my breath
expanding my chest, suddenly I find that I
am not my breath, not my ribs, not my heart
opening, not my feet resting on the ground,
not my legs supporting my weight, not my
arms extending. Suddenly I am a vast
spaciousness. I am the Stillness from which
all things are held.

Chapter Six

The Egoic Governance of Strength Training

Years ago I was training at my gym just outside of Boulder, Colorado. Underneath the high arching ceiling and bright hanging lights I was at the edge of the machine section of my gym sitting on the bench of a seated row machine just a few feet from the coveted water fountain. I had just finished a set of rows followed by back bends off the edge of the bench. As I sat up, my attention shifted from my own training process and fixated upon a trainer with his client two machines down from me. In this moment distractibility governed my experience.

I watched and listened in on a trainer describe his latest ski trip from last weekend with his client. Anger flooded my body. Their conversation continued in an unbroken fashion, just as it might at a coffee shop, although this exchange unfolded during the client's entire working set of leg extensions. The client, mid set, was even adding his own commentary on his lack of skiing this season due to his knee injury. As the set ended they both continued with their conversation. Shortly thereafter the trainer instructed the client to begin another set. The ski conversation continued on and I have no doubt it mutated into a series of what would amount to meaningless tangents as it had largely no meaningful positive impact upon the quality of training performed, at least none that I could see. It was "filler."

I was fuming. This man was supposed to be a professional. What was he getting paid for? Part of me wanted to leap up from my bench and tell them, "Shut up!" I yearned to point out the myriad ways in which the trainer was wasting the client's resources, then to tell the man "Get off that machine, now!" and demonstrate a real working set of leg extensions. I could feel my immense love for the discipline of strength training, and I felt as though these two clowns were pissing on it without any respect. But, for me, this was all my own distraction. As such, I conducted my anger throughout my body as I recalibrated my focus and engagement back into what mattered most. I firmly gripped the handles, lengthened my exhalation, yoked my body and mind back to my central intention and dove back into the fire of my training.

Both my own wandering attention, as well as the immense distractibility demonstrated by trainer and client alike are expressions of the egoic governance of strength training. The ego's distractibility, which is a microcosm of the myth of disengagement at work, is one such way the ego governs strength training. In the moment, hidden behind your activity is a pervasive searching that continually disengages you. Your attention rests briefly on one dimension of training only to be distracted to something else. Your ego is not even clear about what it is looking for most of the time. Anything else will usually suffice.

For me, it was people not respecting the discipline of strength training and my ego fixating upon how it should be engaged and how professionals should conduct themselves with clients. For the trainer, distractibility might have arisen out of his insecurity and uncertainty on how to use the space between him and his client. Perhaps he began to fill this unknown space with habituated social conversations distracting himself from feeling insecure. The client, who was not complaining in the least, might have been somewhat content in distracting his attention from the genuine work of training. In each case, the ego's susceptibility for distraction governed the experience of training.

Recently I was having a conversation with a close friend of mine who has just begun his work as a professional trainer, so he is filled with questions. Coupled with this curiosity he also has immense potential to cut through the egoic fixations of his clients to reveal the deeper core of strength training. We spent some time talking about his client's pervasive desire for novelty. They are wanting new and different exercises to work specific parts of their body. This desire for something, anything, new, leads us to another major way the ego governs strength training. The ego worships novelty.

Take a look at your monthly fitness magazines of any variety and you will see month in and month out, year in and year out, "new" exercises and "new" training programs that get you results fast. Novelty and speed: If you combine the two, you have an addictive combination that grips two of the most powerful egoic desires, which are "Give me something else!" and "Give me something else, fast!"

The ego desires novelty because, no matter what you have right now or where you are, your ego struggles with it and therefore cannot find genuine happiness. Happiness is to be found in something else. The easiest place to look is in something novel. Your ego desires speed because getting out of this (remember from the ego's perspective it does not matter where "this" is) as fast as possible is what the ego most wants. Within the ego's pervasive struggle, it desires to get out of this present situation and into something else, and the faster the better.

As a result, novelty is a common feature in strength training. Personal trainers often specialize in novelty to keep their clients engaged. Many different exercises for training any one part of the body have been developed in response to this need for novelty. Clients, after experiencing one, unconsciously ask for another. Watch someone over time, and you are likely to see them compulsively trying out one new strategy after another. Some literally try something else each set. Others will pick up a new training program each month. Often individuals fail to develop a requisite focus and engagement of any of the strategies they are "trying out" to elicit the physiological adaptations they are searching for. As such it is a common inner dialogue to think to themselves, "Well this isn't working; maybe I'll try that other strategy." Quietly, behind all of this inner chatter, the ego says, "Yes, give me something else." The present strength training paradigm is disengaged from, while the desired happiness and results move again to something over there, something new, something exciting and different to capture the ego's fascination, at least for a little while. This is the ego's compulsive move toward novelty.

Most conventional approaches to strength training, as you may have already started to notice, largely stem from the ego's habituated struggle. A typical example is the intention to lose weight. Struggling with your body image, the way you look and feel, and desiring to have a different weight or set of measurements largely result in your habituation's further grip upon you. Similarly the desire to gain some measure of athletic capacity or to get rid of some weaknesses are often equally governed solely by your habituation's hold on you. The desire to feel good about yourself, to gain more energy, to change your mood or become more healthy are all likely to be fundamentally invested in the ego's desire to get somewhere else. The examples are virtually endless as the ego's most essential process creates tension and struggle continuously.

To be clear, there is nothing intrinsically wrong with these goals. They all possess some degree of truth, elegance and beauty to them. The problem is when these real and alive intentions are hijacked and solely governed by your ego's habituated struggle. When you actually go into the gym and begin strength training from the ego's dictatorship the problem is simple: Habituated struggle is incredibly inefficient at attaining elegant goals that can serve both you and others.

You may start with a sincere desire and aspiration, but soon after you actually begin your training, a broad spectrum of egoic hindrances surface. Perhaps it is a pervasive distractibility as the ego begins to daydream about another part of life or a distracting social exchange with an acquaintance. Maybe the compulsion to do something new and different arises after you witness someone doing an exercise you have never seen before. So, instead of engaging the routine that might actually serve you if you genuinely committed yourself to it, you start tinkering with new exercises. Maybe you begin to experience boredom, which is the ego's way of energetically saying, "I want something else, preferably something more exciting."

Maybe your training has developed into an intensity, vigor and focus that actually can begin to yield the results that you are driven to achieve. In this case one of the ego's most devastating expressions of its habituated struggle tends to show up in your training: the divorce from your embodiment. This egoic pattern is particularly pervasive in strength training and it is perhaps one of the most stunting habituations that limits achievement. Here the ego distances and dissociates from your body's direct and immediate sensations. In this inner distancing you will see the ego's ingrained attachment to comfort. Reach a level of intensity that yields sensations that are not what the ego considers to be "comfortable" and the ego habitually disengages training and divorces its connection with your body in service of comfortability.

In conventional strength training the ego often seeks comfort residing in two points in time. During an exercise, the ego believes that happiness resides when the set is finished. Once you begin your exercise and the sensations of training begin to rise, bringing about a sense of discomfort, your ego projects happiness into the end of the set. Therein lies the gravity of egoic strength training: *stopping*. It does not matter if you are doing pull-ups, dips, squats, bench presses or any other exercise, when your ego is in control and you are caught by the myth of disengagement, you are likely to think about stopping. You may ask yourself, "When should I stop?" and even ponder how great it is going to be once you do stop your set. When your set ends, you will not find happiness with your ego in control. Instead you commonly will be enveloped by the comfortable habituated struggle that covers up your aliveness, engagement and Excellence.

The second period of time your ego often focuses upon is when you have finished your training altogether. Perhaps it is after you have finished a set and you are walking around the gym between exercises that your ego begins to project happiness upon going home, getting to the office or heading to your next commitment. Thus we have the subtle egoic belief running throughout training, "When I am done, I will be happy." While the ego maintains that happiness "resides" in stopping the set, the same process continues once you do stop and happiness is now projected into finishing your training altogether. While your ego is masterful at managing comfort, your ego's habituation is inept at cultivating any real connection with true happiness in your training (or anywhere else in your life).

Outside of seeking these two points in time, routine struggle itself is one of the most comforting experiences for the ego; therefore we will look at the habituated struggle within obligation and desire. These two influential forms of egoically governed strength training are likely to be familiar to you. Stop for a moment and ask your ego, why you train.

When we pose this question and listen into the ego's thought stream, the habitual thought patterns of your conventional mind, you will probably be able to hear these conditioned parts of yourself in some fashion. If you listen in closely you may find one particular expression of your ego's habituation I call "The Shoulds."

"I should be in better shape"
"I should do this because I need to perform better"
"I should improve my athleticism"
"I should do this because its good for me"
"I should because I need to look better"
"I should because I need to do more than ..."
"I should do this because everyone else is"
"I should because my doctor/coach told me to"
"I should because ..."

The ego absolutely loves "should" statements. Whenever you do not genuinely feel like doing some activity, your ego has the relatively easy task of pointing out all the reasons you should indeed do it. Many of the above examples might apply; maybe your ego thinks you should change the way you look or perhaps become more healthy. The opposite is also commonly leveraged by the ego to create struggle: You authentically want to do something, but soon enough you find a plethora of reasons you should not. For example, let us say you have a genuine desire to go for a hike, yet somehow you suddenly find yourself cleaning the bathroom floors instead of going on that hike.

This is the essence of ego. You are split and divided in the moment. Part of you thinks you should, while the other part does not feel like it. When you act from an obligation you may notice that these often reinforce your habituated struggles, thereby strengthening egoic functioning within strength training.

A second egoic thought pattern you may hear as you listen into your own habituated inner dialogue involves the phrase "I have to." Your ego enjoys this strategy because the belief that you "have to" train in order to achieve some worthwhile goal plays nicely into the ego's fundamental rejection of what is here, in its seemingly endless desire to get somewhere else. While most likely your ego is correct in its assertions (you will not achieve various adaptations from *not* training) it nonetheless grabs onto the desired outcomes while resisting the path necessary to achieve those outcomes. Again you are divided. Part of you wants the worthy end "result" yet another part of you resists doing the necessary work, thus you "have to" do the training. Ultimately you will struggle endlessly on this path so long as your functioning remains identified to your ego. Your ego thrives on this struggle and uses this conditioning to perpetuate its influence over your training (and life).

Regardless of whether you train exclusively as a means to accomplish a goal, or feel an obligation to conform to some personal or social norm, you are often reinforcing and entrenching your egoic functioning when you enact the discipline of strength training from the ego's struggle. Whenever you do so you are likely to find yourself manufacturing the myth of disengagement in some form in your training. This illusion maintains, just as it does in the rest of your life, that if you could just get rid of a particular burdening obligation or if you could just achieve some worthy goal and free yourself of the activity of pursuit, only then would you find happiness and a sense of peace.

As habituation unfolds moment to moment, the lie that comfort is the same as happiness often runs rampant in your training. Conventional training's true orientation is comfortability. As you train from ego you will see that you are not actually doing much strength training at all. Physically you may be going through some motions, but mentally and emotionally you are training something else, most notably your habituated negotiation for comfort and the compulsive activity of struggle itself. This is a terribly ineffective way of training, although it is effective at maintaining comfort for your ego. Ultimately egoic forms of strength training are not aimed at happiness, the achievement of your goals, the authentic realization of your larger strength as a human being or your greater Excellence. These are products of something else guiding your strength training. These are born from training to discover and articulate who you are right now. This is something altogether different.

Attunement & Joy: Your Ego's Adversaries

We have seen that much of conventional strength training (and life) is governed by egoic expressions of habituation. To clarify, your *ego* does not want happiness and joy. *You* are drawn to love, happiness and unbounded joy. Ego is drawn to and attached to comfort, not happiness. The ego masquerades within your training with the appearance that it too is in search of happiness and your well-intended goals. A closer inspection often reveals that these experiences and outcomes are directly opposed to the fabric of ego's ongoing struggle. For to genuinely accept the achievement of a worthy goal and to inhabit your true seat of happiness would largely result in the cessation of your ego's habituated struggle.

Conventional training yields comfort, not happiness. Thus we hold the answer to why most people do not love their strength training and why they do not find themselves filled with enjoyment. It is difficult to find those who are ecstatically enjoying the movement of their body and mind in their training because so much of strength training today is governed by the fragmented approaches egoic habituation gives rise to. Instead of euphoric releases upon the completion of a set, we find distance from the direct embodied truth of experience. Rather than open-hearted love, we find the avoidance of what appears to be arduous pain. Instead of conscious liberation, we find dull habituation.

Because the ego is unskilled at cultivating an attunement with the present moment, conventional strength training is infused with an inability to fully participate with the truth of your direct lived experience. Your ego rejects the unconditioned acceptance of the present moment, and with it happiness, along with your greater skillfulness in your training. When attunement with the present moment is replaced by a habituated struggle with the present you become incredibly ineffective and inefficient.

As you are training you must have the strength to pierce through your habituation and attune to the genuine aliveness, energy and flow of your training. You must *practice*. Your Excellence is calling you to refine your greatest capacities from your most essential liberation.

If your heart genuinely wants to increase your performance capacities or change the way you look, beautiful! Just do not attempt to do it by fragmenting your inner organization through struggle. Do not disorganize your energy into opposing and conflicted positions. These approaches actually make no sense when you drop the trance of egoic habituation. Pursue your aims from a greater integration with every facet of your being and then see what and whom you become. This is where true progress is made, where elegance and the larger emergence of your Excellence reside.

Ultimately strength training is a microcosm of the macrocosm of your life. How you train reflects how you live the rest of your life. For the millions trapped in conventional forms of strength training, they are also trapped in the conventional egoic habituations of day-to-day life. As a result, most people go through both their workouts and life wanting something else, desiring something else and rejecting what is right here and now in favor of some imagined future or recaptured past, neither of which actually exists.

Chapter Seven
Your Body-Mind

Thus far we have talked quite a bit about your ego, which, from the perspective taken, has been a mental construct. While this is partially true, it is also leaving out an essential dimension: the body. A more accurate view of both yourself and your ego is to view yourself as a self system[13]. This self system can be most easily summarized as a "body-mind." The ego prefers to view itself as just a mind, a thinking entity. This is for a broad range of reasons; however, at the center, your ego possesses a fear of the body and, ultimately, the body's undeniable connection with death.

The mental constructs your ego employs to define itself have correlative holding patterns in the body. Thus your ego is more accurately represented as a certain mental perspective *and* a particular posture in your body; the two work in concert. It naturally follows then that the most skillful and effective way to work with your ego, and to genuinely transform your training, is to take a more integrated approach and address both the mental and physical dimensions of your ego. You may recall your ego's most basic process is to struggle with what is in the moment. This manifests in your body in a number of ways, the most important of which as it pertains to our discussion is through muscular tension.

Mental Struggle = Muscular Tension

Struggle equals tension. This is the basic formula. Tension in the body creates struggle in the mind; struggle in the mind creates tension in the body. At no time will you ever be struggling with something mentally and at the same time be completely relaxed, open and at peace in your body. The two are intimately linked.

Here is the central point for you. Your ego has a certain range of tension in which it flourishes. Too little tension dissolves the basic struggle with what is and thus threatens the ego's fundamental position. Your ego's lower boundary is where your ego habitually introduces struggle and tension. Similarly, too much tension starts to rub up against the ego's attachment to being comfortable. At a certain level of intensity your body-mind must become incredibly centered and focused in the present moment. As a result your conventional construction of past and future start to break down into an immediacy of the present moment in which your ego's grip on control dissolves. The ego's upper boundary is found where ego habitually disengages from high levels of tension.

As you might have guessed, the ego employs a beautifully rich array of strategies to regulate your body-mind and keep you in its perceived "safe zone" where your ego can comfortably operate and control your life and your course of action. As the tension in the body progressively decreases, your ego will introduce struggle on some level. Why? At a certain level of relaxation or Surrender the present moment emerges as the center of your experience and your ego thus loses its sense of control, and fundamentally the identity of your ego starts to dissolve[14].

Similarly, as tension increases and starts to nudge up against your ego's comfortable range of functioning, it will develop strategies to diminish the tension and struggle in your body-mind. Once again, at a certain level, which tends to differ from one person to the next, your ego's autonomy and foundation of identity start to dissolve and pass away, as the intensity of the tension and struggle progressively enters the immediacy of the present moment.

To give a quick example of how your ego will regulate these two boundaries, let us take a look at an exercise: the bench press. As you lift the bar from the stand, you begin your first repetition. Your mind notices the weight as something familiar, and your body-mind follows the form you have trained yourself to execute. As this set progresses you might start comparing your strength to previous workouts. Perhaps you start to tell yourself "I am a little bit weaker today." The sensations in your chest, shoulders and arms start to increase as you do a couple more repetitions and you start to evaluate yourself. "Can I get to twelve repetitions?" You know your goal is twelve, but now, as the intensity grows, part of you wants to quit. Perhaps you are telling yourself, "This might be good enough," as you begin to press up your ninth repetition.

Suddenly you are standing next to the bench realizing that somewhere along the course of your last few reps you fell into an unconscious state and hit autopilot. You know you got eleven, but you did not make a conscious choice to stop at eleven.

This is a classic example of "checking out." Intensity gets too high, and poof, you disappear and immediately a habitual pattern cuts in and ends the set for you. You have just hit your upper ego boundary. This is not just a psychological boundary, although your mind has a huge role in growing and expanding this boundary upwards. You also need to develop your nervous system, musculature and joints to be able to conduct the increased bandwidth of intensity these extra repetitions require when you do go for that twelfth repetition, and perhaps the thirteenth, in our example.

Let us say you are going to practice a relaxation technique after a set to optimize your recovery and prepare yourself for the next set. You take a seat on the bench and close your eyes. You start to relax your muscles, breathe deeply and rhythmically into your belly and begin witnessing everything that is arising without trying to change anything. There is a vitality swimming through your body-mind that is refreshingly enjoyable. After a few more breaths your mind may start to wander off to random thoughts about various parts of your life. As soon as this occurs and you stop remaining vividly aware of your relaxation you have just hit your lower ego boundary. Your ego needed to introduce some "doing" into an activity that is fundamentally a "being" exercise, something extra. The moment in its bare presence contains no struggle, no problem and thus your ego needs to generate tension. Strength training as an Integral Practice works on these two basic ego boundaries.

Let us explore one more example of how your ego's upper boundary is engaged and challenged within each set of exercises in your training. Let us say you are going to do three sets of squats. Each set can be used to do two key tasks. First, each set can be used to expand your ego's upper boundary if a sufficient amount of energy is conducted, engaged with and concentrated into each repetition of each set. Secondly, as you learn to navigate your ego's strategies to keep you in your "safe zone" you can cultivate an essential seat of awareness that intrinsically extends beyond your ego. That is to say, as the intensity increases, the repetitions go up, and your habituated sense of self attempts to take control of the process, you simply witness your ego instead of compulsively acting on it.

The meditator whose mind has wandered off into thinking about some aspect of his or her life and the strength trainer doing squats who has wandered from the present moment share the same basic process. The stability of the body-mind dissolves and the present moment is no longer properly held. The meditator may come back to the present moment with a number of points of focus: the breath, posture or a mantra. Similarly the strength trainer comes back to the present moment through focusing on breath, form, or sensation (or perhaps what is being avoided most, which typically takes the form of intense vibrational frequencies in the musculature caused by the contraction and exertion of your muscles.)

Through this process the exclusive identification with your ego dissolves, and a more expansive sense of self immediately emerges to inhabit a broader context of experience. Within the most intense sets it is common for a spaciousness to emerge. In the midst of a storm of vibrations throughout your musculature, a stillness and expansiveness can emerge as part of your experience. This spaciousness is not checking out, but rather it is the liberation from the confines of the ego. This space found within intensity is often experienced as unmoving, resourced and attuned meaning that within the intensity of movement simultaneously you feel the inside of a stillness that provides more energy for engaging precisely what is.

As you start to engage the parts of yourself that transcend the ego, of which this is just one, your performance on the more relative and conventional levels will often improve, sometimes dramatically. You will be tapping your larger potential as a human being and learning how to manifest this transcendent seat into your body-mind. As you learn to master this process, you will develop access to a new reservoir of power, strength, energy, focus and so on. These additional resources enable you to supersede what you were capable of doing within the bounds of your ego and your historical conditioning, which is largely aimed at turning away from intensity as you approach your ego's upper boundary.

Your second threshold is the lower ego boundary (the point at which the ego introduces struggle because the self does not hold enough resistance with the present moment). If there is one thing the ego truly resists beyond pain, it is Surrender. Think about it, who do you know that is really good at Surrendering to what is going on in the present moment while being relaxed, centered and at peace within the most stressful situations? Chances are you do not know many people like this. Strength training can explicitly develop these skills for you, although these are skills your ego fundamentally cannot possess. So, if you want to adopt, grow and master the skill of true Surrender and recovery, you will have to shift your self system's "center of gravity" beyond the ego's habituation.

Now you might ask yourself: "How does strength training activate and engage this recovery, relaxation and Surrender?" And this is an excellent question as it is not immediately apparent. Certainly working with your lower ego boundary is not as obvious as is expanding your ego's upper boundary. Let us look at how strength training can help you expand your range of functioning using our example of doing three sets of squats.

As you expand, grow and, at times, transcend your ego's upper boundary during the squats, in between each set you will be intentionally recovering, relaxing and Surrendering. It is in the space between your lifts where the growth and expansion of your lower ego boundary occurs. Conventional forms of strength training do not generally employ this dimension. Instead, it is common for people to have distracting conversations, watch TV, space out or fill their time with other ego-driven distractions. If you are focused on growing through your training you may myopically focus upon the expansion of the upper ego boundary. This is another form of egoic distraction from your body-mind's optimal recovery for authentic peak levels of execution that reside beyond the territory of your egoic struggle.

Surrender, relaxation and recovery are all difficult to master and employ strategically between each set throughout your training. Primarily because it is something you cannot do. Rather it is something you must allow to happen, and this often takes a lot of practice. Particularly if you want to master allowing your ego's controlling grip to dissolve away, which gives you access to your most potent source of rejuvenation and recovery.

Later on we will discuss the specific techniques you can use to grow, expand and transcend your ego's upper and lower boundaries. However it is important to note here that it is through engaging the present moment that you make true progress and by which you recover, relax and rejuvenate your body-mind. There is no disengaging involved in this process.

To skillfully work in the most efficient and effective way in order to transform your training and articulate the greater sphere of your Excellence, you must move beyond the fragmented perspective of being an ego that possesses a body. You are a body-mind and your ego manifests through both mental and physical phenomena. Your training requires that you expand both your upper and lower boundaries so that your egoic functioning is more open, fluid and dynamic. As your ego is cultivated, your capacity to remain attuned to and engaged with the present moment is improved. Furthermore, at the heart of transforming your training is the call to enact your training from beyond the compulsive habituated struggle of your ego. It is from this liberated seat of functioning that the transformation, performance and Excellence that you seek is brought to fruition. This is the doorway through which all else follows in your training and evolving unfolding.

Chapter Eight
Engaging Wholeheartedly

As you will see, each moment in your training is an invitation for wholehearted engagement. Habitually the ego divides and fragments your energy into a persistent struggle. Engaging wholeheartedly is an ever present opportunity to step into a realm of wakeful presence that is liberated from egoic contraction. Instead of turning away from the complete embodiment of your aliveness, this gesture of full engagement faces your embodied aliveness openly. Before theoretically investigating this gesture of engaging wholeheartedly let me offer the following example of leg presses from my experience with training. This is one window into the type of engagement we now turn our attention to.

I am on a mat next to the leg press machine located dead center in the weight training facility at my gym. My body-mind stretches between a massive painted concrete pillar on my right, reaching up toward the high white celling, and the gray leg press machine on my left. It is loaded with about as much weight as the machine can possibly hold; somewhere between 1200 and 1300 pounds of black iron rest quietly waiting to exert their force upon me. My body-mind is yoking into Eka Pada Rajakapotasana, or what is more commonly known as "pigeon pose" in yoga. Pigeon is particularly good at opening the hips, which is the primary focus in this moment.

My hips sink into the mat, my tailbone reaches downward and my heart and crown lift upward as my shoulder blades melt down my back. I release my exhalation, lengthening my out-breath as my body deepens the stretch in my hips. I am centered, stable and inhabiting the intense immediacy of sensation in my body-mind. I feel amazing. I slowly draw out of this asana, making my way to my feet where I shake out my legs as I pace toward the mirrors and then back to the leg press a few times. My attention is open and relaxed. For a precious moment all seeking ceases. I am going "nowhere." I am present. Breath infuses me with pleasure. As I turn toward the leg press my attention merges into preparations for my next set.

I can feel my intention permeating what seems to be all of me. My heart's awareness circles to include and participate with the full scope of my direct embodied experience. The bliss from breathing and opening my hips is circulating through my body-mind. My quadriceps are flushed with blood, they feel weaker yet more alive from my previous sets. Consciousness has joined with the muscle tissue itself. I feel a subtle resistance within my mind's habituated script. Softly my conditioning advocates for "taking it easy," which more specifically means for me "Stop as soon as possible." Yet, I also feel my heart's movement toward the unconditioned inclusion of intensity. This is the larger truth of my experience. Something timeless inside of me wants an aliveness that is brought to the fore with exertion. I yearn for it unmediated and raw. My breathing quickens, my hands make gentle fists as I begin to hit my hips and quads.

My body-mind is open and playful to what is present in my experience. I am attuned and wakeful as I step over the sturdy beams of the machine and sit down into the seat. I shift my sit bones around subtly to anchor my hips into the firm cushion of the seat and to find the perfect alignment in my spine. I feel this sense of perfection resonate through me when I find it. Next my feet shift around the leg press to find the position that feels right. I even wiggle my toes and shift my feet in my shoes to place my feet into a perfection inside my shoes. The world is falling away now. There is no sound outside my breath. No one else is in the gym. No work. No distraction. My body-mind focuses on 40 repetitions. Today I am training strong range partials, which are quick, explosive movements through the strongest range of movement. While I am still, I can feel the pressing currents of energy moving in my still body.

I breathe in forcefully. Air, life and energy rush into me as I conduct this breath into my belly. A fluid tension holds my core tight as this pressure of breath and abdominal muscles adds stability to my spine. I explode into the weight and release the safety handles away from my sides.

My hands swiftly grab hold of the handle bars as I strongly pull downward further anchoring my hips into place. Repetitions are fast yet controlled, and I focus upon moving the weight as quickly as possible and then controlling the weight back down to my starting point. My breath and movement are flowing as one. Forcefully I breathe into my belly and explosively I exhale to empty all the air precisely at the top of my leg press.

Here at the top I am careful not to lock out my knees thus transferring more energy into my leg muscles. Each cresting movement involves me totally extending my energy out through my extended legs, and years of practice swiftly draws a gentle bend in the knees to catch the weight's descent into the musculature. The pressure of this weight is aliveness pressing into me. A few repetitions into the set, my attention is scanning throughout my body: hips, spine, knees, ankles, right hamstring. I am feeling through all my major joints and muscles making sure all systems and structures feel safe.

As the reps increase my breathing expands to take in more air. My movements become more precise. My attention settles down into the direct immediacy of sensation primarily in my quadriceps, gluteus, hamstrings and calf muscles. My whole body feels as though it is breathing. With each repetition the sensations in my working muscles increase in warm, alive vibrations.

At around 20 repetitions my chin drops and my body and mind fracture, with vibrations in my body perceived as pain in my mind. I feel my conditioned response to stop, to fall effortlessly into what is most comfortable. Two things are happening in my ego: my mind is fabricating a story about how painful this is and my ego is imagining how stopping is going to feel good. I quickly lift my chin, aligning my spine and witness this habituated movement toward comfort in my body-mind. I feel my heart's inclusion of all of my experience and I consciously breathe deeper. Pressing into my feet I attune to what is precisely here in my experience. I align my knees and plunge back into the immediacy of sensation. I feel the movement of my unconditioned heart. This precious source pours outward filling seemingly everything that I am. My attention naturally and effortlessly turns right into precisely what my habituation resists the most; the pain resonating in my legs begins to merge with a perceived aliveness.

I feel my face contracting and contorting as I press again and again into the weight. I release as much tension in my face as I am able and conduct this energy into my legs. Spontaneously my eyes become completely still and my body relaxes within the intensity of movement. The sensations in my legs are vibrating at an incredible rate. They are hot, painful and anything but comfortable, but in the relaxation in my face, as my eyes become utterly still and my body finds a looseness amidst these leg presses, the vibration, heat and pain join with pleasure. It is subtle at first, but with each repetition the ecstatic bliss grows and flowers into more and more of my body-mind.

I am grunting yet somehow moaning at the same time. I have let go of any counting. I breathe, press into the weight and engage. Repetition after repetition my attention fluidly plays within the intensity of sensation. Suddenly I feel a space inside of all of my sensation; it is black and empty. Within the intense vibration there is a sensation of incredible stillness. My attention moves toward this paradox and I feel a pregnant spaciousness on the inside of these waves of pleasure and pain. I have stopped pressing into the machine and instead, a pressing movement is doing me, although I am not on autopilot. I am completely present, centered and resting in a peacefulness.

My heart is breaking open into a love of this singular moment. I feel the fullness of each moment and almost simultaneously grieve the loss as this moment dies and births a new full, rich and amazing experience of life. Seemingly every facet of my being focuses into this single movement. This is but one example, one "taste," of engaging wholeheartedly.

Engaging wholeheartedly involves three elements: intention, attunement and engagement. Intention is the first of two inner movements necessary for engaging wholeheartedly. Your intention is an aligning of your willpower and a clarifying of your attention which prepares you to take action. This can all be done without actually moving your body, thus it is an inner movement. The second inner movement, attunement, cultivates a relationship with what is present. Finally, engagement brings outer action as your body-mind takes action. To engage wholeheartedly you must yoke together and integrate these three elements into your training. We will begin by exploring intention and walk our way through each of the central components of engaging wholeheartedly.

Engaging wholeheartedly is in direct contrast with the ego's habituated struggle. The ego almost perpetually divides itself into conflicting positions. As such, training with the ego in control involves a fragmented approach where struggle governs the process and outcome of your training. This can be thought of as "engaging partially" or "engaging halfheartedly." The starting point for unraveling the ego's grip on your sense of self and how you train (as well as how you conduct yourself in your life as a whole) is intention.

Strength training as an Integral Practice always begins with the inner movement of intention, but not just any intention. Some intentions are solely ruled and operated by the ego's basic stance toward the present moment. As explored in Chapter Six some common guiding intentions for practitioners first stepping into strength training are to lose weight, improve performance or change the way they look in some fashion amongst a host of other valuable aspirations. These intentions are, generally speaking, governed by the ego's struggle. They are often married to the desire to be different, to get somewhere else or perhaps be something that at least right now you are not.

Engaging strength training exclusively from these intentions often results in the entrenching of your ego's functioning. This is problematic because while these desires are often well-intended, they are governed by the ego's less structured and less pragmatic level of functioning. Let me repeat this because it is extremely important. Your ego, when compared to your integrated body-mind that originates beyond the ego, is *less structured, less pragmatic, less effective and less efficient* in the gym and in the world. Thus these well intended side-effects of training lead many astray from the start. They reinforce the ego's incredibly inefficient habituated struggles. These conventional intentions are not the originating source of an Integral Practice in strength training.

The primary intention that can liberate you from conventional approaches to strength training is, in part, what I call engaging wholeheartedly. This intention establishes the bridge upon which you can cross from ego-driven training to a discipline driven from a more expansive sense of self, a dimension of you that is liberated from your ego's habituation. This transition beyond the ego's control is an essential quality necessary if an intention is to give birth to a genuine Integral Practice where all of your major faculties are engaged in the direct immediacy of your training.

Understood properly, the intention to engage wholeheartedly steers you toward embracing and participating with who you are in your full and liberated embodiment right here and now. Training feels distinctly different from this perspective. Depending on what training methodology is employed the same external physiological changes occur: weight loss, muscle gain, adaptations in power or endurance and changes in physical appearance. The difference with an intention that is not governed by struggle is twofold. First, your interior faculties (mental, emotional and spiritual capacities) are more actively engaged in your training. Second, external development (the physiological and energetic adaptations and refinements) typically unfolds with greater efficiency. Ultimately though, your life fundamentally depends upon the clarity of your intention to grow beyond the ego's habituated struggle.

Now as you read this last sentence your ego might say "My life does not depend upon committing to a path that leads beyond the ego!" From the ego's vantage point your life is going to go on just fine. You will have ups and downs, you will learn in the process and both fail and achieve along the way, but in no way does your life depend upon committing to a "trans-egoic" path. And your ego's perspective is correct. It is perfectly valid, but only within its own conventional worldview. However, from a deeper perspective your life depends upon a committed decision to forge a path beyond ego.

From the ego's perspective on life, happiness, success and contentment all reside in obtaining something in the future. After all, the relationship to the present moment is fundamentally overlooked by the ego because the next moment is always coming. So it makes more sense to focus on the future, to plan, prepare, control, and manage the best the ego can. This is largely a conditioned response to your personal history. This is most certainly a valid perspective, but there is a *more* valid perspective emerging that integrates the forward-looking pragmatic functioning and goes beyond the ego's constrained pragmatism.

This moment is the entirety of your life.

Stop and read the above line again. Take the time to let it sink in a bit and open the process of shifting beyond your conventional means of meaning-making. This moment is your life. Life is all right here.

Your ego says, "Yes, but I've got more time coming to me." And from a more conventional standpoint this is true (unless you are knowingly or unknowingly taking your last breath.)

What does exist though? What ever really exists? It is this present moment. It is this word that you are reading right now. It is this breath, this thought, this intention happening right now. The past did exist but it is gone. The future will come. Neither of which is your life right now.

Your life depends on a commitment to enact a path that leads you beyond your ego.

As you read the above sentence, are you starting to interpret "your life" as the present moment? Or are you still thinking about your life as the string of past, present and future moments leading toward something. One perspective is shifting beyond your ego. The other is of reinforcing your ego's gripping worldview. One perspective excludes and struggles with the present moment while another includes the past, present and future. The ego's vantage point on life is indeed useful; however, it is also incredibly limited and therefore should not be overvalued at the expense of other perspectives that may be more inclusive and effective.

Perhaps more than any other thing in life, you (not your ego) need to make a clear decision and commitment to train yourself in order to continually live beyond your ego's habituated approach to life. Just as there is an entire world beyond the reach of the child's grasp, so too is there an entire world beyond the ego's grasp. There is a larger perspective to be experienced and from which to animate your training (and life). This more integrative vantage point standing beyond ego is what allows you to live your life more fully, with greater happiness, peace and success. Ultimately the quality of your life depends upon your relationship to the present moment.

It follows that the quality and depth of your life, the degree of vitality coursing through your heart and body-mind in this breath, depends upon your intention and commitment to follow a path that leads beyond your habituated ego.

Your more integrative perspective understands the immense importance of the present moment. As you start to settle into understanding this moment and how it is intrinsically tied to your happiness, vitality and purpose of your life, you will start to feel that this is truly the only moment you have (or from another perspective, the only moment that holds you). The more you shift beyond your egoic perspective the stronger and more transparent this simple truth becomes.

Often in response to this intuition your ego will create a sense of urgency and panic. While your ego has good intentions, ultimately this sense of impulsive urgency continues to disconnect you from this moment and the source of your vitality. As you awaken, enliven and grow, your ego will attempt to possess the moment. As a result, instead of being possessed and enlivened by the moment, inspired by the now, you will slowly die and shift back into a lower frequency.

Engaging wholeheartedly can liberate you from these lower frequencies inherent in egoic functioning, although this is not a certainty. It is possible for your ego to co-opt this intention to extend or maintain its control. As such, you must properly understand this intention to move your functioning beyond your ego's habituated power, control and limited autonomy. Two common misunderstandings of the intention to engage wholeheartedly are as follows:

1. *Destination*: Engaging wholeheartedly is not a destination that you will arrive at in the future and it is certainly not a destination where you will experience only the positive attributes your ego appears to habitually search for.

It is most simply a starting point and orientation. Engaging wholeheartedly has one location: the present moment. Its simplicity is what retains its power. This guiding intention is the full engagement of your faculties into what is here and now without discrimination. Manufacturing this intention into some expectation, overt or subtle in nature, fragments your engagement and entrenches the ego's struggle.

2. *No Struggle*: Engaging wholeheartedly is not a state (or destination) in which you have released all struggle.

The belief that when you are strength training you should not struggle with what is happening is a misperception and misunderstanding of this guiding intention. This is the result of the intention to engage wholeheartedly being hijacked by the ego. With the ego in control struggle is being further established between struggling and not struggling. While the ego may have been forced to adopt a more subtle strategy, you still remain within the bonds of the ego's conditioned grip.

While you may experience short periods or states in which your ego's habituated struggle disappears temporarily, the larger journey is one that is, face to face, participating with your ego's habituation with great attunement. Instead of confronting your ego *from* ego, or bringing more struggle to the struggle that is already present, engaging wholeheartedly involves participating with ego from the dimension of yourself that is fundamentally committed to not struggling. When you genuinely participate with your ego from the dimension of you that is the center of Being itself, there is no need to try (struggle) to get rid of struggle, for to do so would fracture the integrity of your presence in the moment. If you are trying to eliminate anything in your training, rest assured that your ego is likely at the helm.

Chapter Nine
The Role of Discipline

Discipline, from a conventional standpoint, is the practice of training someone to obey a set of rules or code of conduct using punishment to correct disobedience. This is not the most uplifting perspective, however it does embody much of our egoic assumptions about discipline. If you do something wrong, something that does not fit into what your parents, social circle or society at large expects or values, you will be disciplined in a variety of ways. Later on in life you will probably deliver this punishment to yourself through your own inner dialogue in an attempt to self-correct your behavior in the world.

For example, in seventh grade I tried out a season of wrestling for my middle school's boys team. I wrestled the 112-pound weight class; the only problem was I weighed exactly 112 pounds. My coach at the time disciplined his team to make our respective weight classes. Some people did not have to worry, others like myself had the problem of being a growing boy with the clear expectation that I would not gain even a single pound. It was fairly simple—if you wanted to wrestle you had to wrestle in the weight class the coach gave you. Gain weight and you would watch instead of wrestle. Conventional discipline left me sitting at my grandmother's dinner table over Christmas passing on seconds while I was still hungry. In my head was my coach telling his team to keep their weight in check over Christmas break.

Another similar conventional view says discipline is a controlled behavior —a "training," if you will—that tries to produce a specific character or pattern of behavior. Generally speaking this training is assumed to produce, or at least be aimed at producing, moral character or personal development in a particular valued direction. For example, your parents might have disciplined you to always make your bed when you got up in the morning, or to be truthful and respectful when speaking to adults. Perhaps a company might discipline their work force with a policy around being late to work or they might offer incentives to complete additional training that is likely to improve on-the-job performance.

As you might have guessed, while this conventional perspective of discipline is indeed valuable and is important for the development of the ego, we are going to be taking a closer look at discipline. We are going to look at the type of discipline required to move beyond your ego. To do so we will start by looking at one of the roots of the word discipline.

Tracing the word discipline back into its Middle English and Latin past we come across the word from which it emerged. Disciple generally means someone who receives instruction from another. *Another* is not just anyone, though. Historically this "another" refers to following a teacher, leader or philosophy. Perhaps the most common example of this in the West is Jesus' disciples. It is here with the word disciple that we find the beginnings of a post-conventional perspective on discipline.

An important aspect of becoming a disciple is how she is not chosen by the teacher or leader (and certainly not chosen by a philosophy), but rather the disciple makes the choice to receive instruction from the teacher or leader. This is quite different from the conventional perspective of discipline in which your ego was at least partially shaped and formed. For example, to a large extent you did not choose the particular upbringing your parents gave you. Instead, it was given to you. This is especially the case early on in life as you passively received your parents' rearing practices, cultural norms and social expectations.

Discipline, as we are to use the term, includes this key element of choice. Discipline, just like disciple, involves a conscious choice to fully engage in a path, instruction and/or teaching. Discipline as we are framing it then holds the ability to lead your largely conventional sense of self and life into something much greater.

Of Necessity

In terms of making lasting, sustainable change in your life, discipline is an absolute necessity. Whether you are working on completing a college degree or want to anchor your everyday experience beyond your conventional sense of self, you must have discipline. The same holds true for liberating your training from the habituation of your ego. Discipline is a necessity.

Shifting beyond the ego requires a discipline that is not resting on or dependent upon your egoic wants and desires. You must choose to enact and engage your path regardless of how you feel in a more conventional sense. For example, you may be tired and not feel like training. From your ego's vantage point you might be drained and overcommitted. None of this matters to the strength of your post-conventional discipline. Feeling drained or perhaps unmotivated are often major obstacles to training for the ego. This is because your ego's basic struggle thrives within the tension between your action and your feelings. Your ego's habituation maintains that it only wants to do what it *feels* like doing. When this conditioning arises you may find yourself rehearsing, "I feel like being social with my friends instead of training today," "I think I'm going to sleep in so I'm more rested for my day ahead," or "I'm going to watch a movie this evening instead of going to the gym." Underneath all of these positions is the subtle feeling of not wanting to engage training. When these are habitually followed, precious time to practice disappears and with it more and more rehearsal of the same continues onward, headed nowhere in particular.

What is on the menu? My ego would like more of the same, please.

In contrast, your larger sense of self moves beyond habituated thoughts and feelings with ease. When you inhabit and act from the part of you that is liberated, your habituated thoughts and feelings are objects arising in your consciousness and not arising as the subjective seat of your identity. When this happens you are no longer exclusively governed by the habituation unfolding in your body-mind. Instead of the conditioned agenda to align your feelings and your actions, your liberated embodiment is willing to feel through the full spectrum of emotions, feelings and sensations and act with great clarity and consideration. From this larger integrated perspective and embodiment you are able to take the course of action that actually serves your larger intelligence and Excellence. Instead of your egoic preferences collapsing around what your ego prefers to feel and prefers to avoid feeling, your liberated intelligence can navigate your training and life with greater skill.

For example, when you are tired and you do not feel like training in a more conventional sense, your liberated discipline to engage in your practice carries precisely this into your training. The direct immediacy of tiredness and resistance is felt throughout your body-mind and conducted into your training. There is no denial and rejection of this part of your experience; there is complete space to feel tired and resistant to your training while the larger more liberated dimension of yourself engages your training wholeheartedly. The full spectrum of your experience is simply part of the path to be worked with and engaged, not covertly or overtly denied, avoided and/or manipulated. As such, the territory of feelings and habituated preferences are no longer subtly or overtly attempting to govern your actions, behaviors and sense of self.

Through consistent engagement, strength training becomes a strong, resilient and dynamic vehicle for growth. It becomes a reservoir for passionate engagement with your training and life. Along with the intention to engage wholeheartedly, strength training can become one of your most effective vehicles for stepping beyond your habituated way of being in the world.

Without an intentional discipline to unfold your ongoing development you will remain largely stuck in your egoic sense of self, training and the life that naturally follows. Occasionally you will have glimpses beyond your ego; however, your "center of gravity" will remain encumbered in your ego's constant struggle. As each moment is grappled with, life's larger freedom, spaciousness and possibility pass you by and your functioning is ensnared in less pragmatic, less structured and less intentional engagement with the activities that tangibly and practically expand your capacity to serve both yourself and the world around you.

The Risk of Discipline

While discipline is a necessity, it also carries great risk. First, anything that you do repeatedly has a tendency to become automatic and unconscious. When any activity becomes entirely automatic you fall asleep. When you stop consciously choosing, your conditioned history takes over and you cease to practice. When you slip back into autopilot your "center of gravity" takes hold and off "you" go, although "you" in your most authentic sense are not really there. Your training (and life) becomes largely the activity of your historically conditioned patterns playing themselves out, all the while your more authentic sense of self remains dormant. You merely repeat yourself. Each time practice stops the dominos are pushed in the predetermined (or largely predetermined) direction of your ego's habituation. Excellence in any real living sense is dead.

Secondly, discipline is actually something the ego loves and thrives on, and thus it introduces another serious risk. Just as your ego loves to hijack intention, so does your ego love to co-opt and manipulate discipline through the ego's struggle. Discipline provides something for your ego to struggle with. Why? True discipline is something that your ego will never possess, thus it is the perfect project to take up, work on and ultimately use as an excuse to keep things the same. Sure your ego masquerades as wanting the various types of benefits strength training has to offer, but ultimately your ego is more invested in struggling with the path to get there. And thus we come to a common story line the ego repeats: "I don't possess enough discipline." Regardless how this is said, feel into how your own ego may rehearse this message.

If you allow your sense of autonomy and control to be dictated by your ego you will heighten and exacerbate your ego's struggle with discipline. Just as with the ego's desire to hijack the intention to engage wholeheartedly, it is worth your time to keep an eye on any sense of struggle that arrises in conjunction with your discipline.

Your ego will struggle in many different ways, however watch for the following tell-tale signs that your ego is in command.

• Watch for your mind rehearsing: "I should strength train..."

"Should" always implies an obligation, oftentimes given to you by someone else who has been or is influential in your life. As we explored the "I should's" in Chapter Six, typically the "should" stems from your inner division of one part of you feeling like you do not want to train for one reason or another while another part of you insists that you should indeed go train. "Should" is often a divided starting point where your ego is in control. Slow down, return to your core intention to engage wholeheartedly and step into your training anew. Division tends to yield more division while integration has a gravity toward greater integration, and thus your discipline, truly giving all of yourself to your practice, moves in concert with your orienting intention.

• Watch for your mind rehearsing: "I have to strength train if ... ."

Having to do something implies that you are trying to get somewhere else which is often, although not always, rooted in your habituated egoic desires. Remember, there is absolutely nothing wrong with wanting to get somewhere else, yearning for some greater expression of yourself or desiring to change a dimension of yourself as long as it is born from your larger engagement and inclusion of yourself and your faculties. Divorcing yourself from the present moment and the larger truth of who you are through struggle is not a sustainable, effective or proficient strategy to refine yourself and your training. As a result, discipline that is wed to having to get somewhere else is inefficient at best and can be harmful to your integrity at worst. Join your desires and inspiration to change, grow and evolve with your larger integration of and engagement with the full sphere of your direct experience as it arises moment to moment.

• Watch for your mind's tendency to "want to" do something.

Even if you have a desire and a "want" to engage with your discipline your ego is often subtly trying to attain or maintain control. Most likely your ego wants an enjoyable experience, preferably one that can be replicated in some fashion. Wanting to train is a fantastic dimension to stabilize your discipline, but the desire to get something enjoyable out of your training will eventually become an obstacle as you move from egoically governed training to a genuine seat of liberation as you engage in your training. With wanting comes a subtle agenda to experience some expectation. While this desire often holds more congruence in your body-mind than, say, the more overt split of "the shoulds" there is often still a subtle struggle happening here as well. This anticipation and investment in an enjoyable expectation unplugs your true liberated engagement of the present moment. As such, when you notice yourself wanting to train the prescription is to slow down, open your attention to what is happening in the moment and return to the intention to engage wholeheartedly.

Ultimately your discipline and path are committed to improving the quality and depth of your training. Instead of using discipline as a place to struggle, use your discipline as an opportunity to inhabit the spiritual faculty within you that is unconditionally committed to non-struggle. Again, non-struggle is not an extension of egoic activity in which the ego attempts to get rid of struggle.

Your true discipline is a giving of yourself to your training. This involves, at its center, a complete sacrifice of your egoic sense of control. This offering is a release that is necessary if you are to know with your own experience your most liberated seat of consciousness. Without discipline this release is extremely rare. While you may experience openings and various expansions beyond your ego's habituation, your greatest liberation is much more profound and thus much more challenging to recognize than these transitory states that come and go. Your heart's desires and your obligations are not abandoned unless they prove to be false to your larger integrity.

Surface desires, fleeting inspirations and transitory distractions are purified in your discipline and sacrifice. As a result, that which is surface joins with the depth of truth resonating in your Being. What is fleeting becomes stable and consistent dimensions of your congruent evolving expressions of your body-mind's Becoming. What was at first a transitory distraction drawing you further and further into habituation becomes a beacon inviting you to participate with the larger truth of your embodied liberation.

Discipline is of absolute necessity for you to transform your training and to give birth to the emergent Excellence that comes to life through your unique body-mind. The structure and boundaries of a respected discipline, one that you have fully given and devoted yourself to, enables you to cut through your conditioned egoic stance that dominates and commands your training and life. As your Excellence calls for more of you, discipline stands firmly within your practice as a vehicle to help you transform, evolve and articulate your ever emergent strength.

Chapter Ten
Novel Emergence
& Your Path To Mastery

Development has been an implicit foundation for our discussion thus far. Our exploration of the purpose of life as well as how you can transform your training has been embedded in a developmental context. The consideration of the refinement of faculties through practice, how Excellence can be enacted with greater skill and how you can genuinely give yourself to the practice of strength training through discipline all have pointed to a developmental move beyond conventional ways of being and functioning. Additionally, the inspection of egoic modes of training and our exploration of the freedom from ego's habituation enabling you to go beyond ego, as well as the ability to discern between the conditioned struggle toward a presupposed future happiness and your genuine movement as happiness all involve significant shifts in development.

Moving forward we will be exploring developmental possibilities in greater detail as it pertains to your capacity to engage in the art of strength training. As such, we will take a closer look at what it means to develop, to set an explicit foundation for the path ahead. Development, evolution and growth are all terms pointing at the same underlying process where you transcend previous limitations, create novelty, expand your faculties and generate greater integrative capacity. These four dimensions of human development interpenetrate one another and together comprise what it means to develop.

Thus far we have been working with two broad developmental stages, one governed by egoic habituation and the second liberated from such conventions. Thus our exploration has returned again and again to supporting one central developmental shift: moving beyond ego. Step out of struggle and into a greater participation with aliveness. The unconscious and unquestioned loyalty to your conditioned egoic struggles has been the developmental starting point for our exploration of strength training. For most people, their first two to three decades of life have been spent establishing, reifying and reinforcing their ego's habituated ways of being and functioning in the world. This is itself an important developmental movement from pre-egoic functioning. This establishment of the ego culminates into what psychologists often call the individuated autonomous ego. This is what many consider to be conventional adulthood.

While many people cease to develop beyond these conventions, human development does stretch far beyond our culture's conventions and average modes of functioning[15]. As development shifts beyond ego a new way of being and functioning emerges. As we have been discussing, habituated struggles are no longer exclusively identified with. That is to say your subjective experience is not subsumed by these deep-seated struggles arising moment to moment. You cease to be the immediacy of your habituated struggles. And therefore ego is no longer the organizing and controlling facility of who you are. What was once your subjective immersion becomes an object within experience that can now be mediated, managed or negotiated with. Instead of *being* the struggle with the direct immediacy of sensation in your body-mind while training, you *have* struggle arising as an object within your now larger self. After this developmental shift, you have been liberated from struggle. Struggle is now a part of your experience, not the context for all of your experience. The novel emergence of this developmental shift is the space that has been created within yourself. In this case it is a space that is interwoven with a faculty that is non-struggling. The novelty of non-struggling space expands your faculties by bringing forth a greater possibility for more choice. Habituated activity is an option, no longer a compulsive necessity. As the self becomes larger (both struggle and non-struggle arise inside of the self) the integrative capacity available also grows. This means that what is able to be included as an object in experience expands. A greater number and diversity of objects can be included with greater flexibility for how to relate and enact. Within the space beyond struggle you can hold more. Your capacity for consideration, discernment and skillful engagement increases. This is, in part, what it means to develop beyond ego.

This brings us to a more refined developmental approach to strength training. It is this work's basic premise that your capacity to engage with the discipline of strength training moves through a developmental sequence. As your engagement of strength training transforms the practice itself, what you are actually doing and participating with also grows in developmental complexity. You grow and what you do grows alongside you. Strength training can therefore be used as a vehicle to transform your self along with a broad spectrum of your faculties. Additionally, if employed properly, Body-Mind-Moment Training can be used to help facilitate some of the highest levels of maturity we presently know of.

We are going to look at one particular developmental model for strength training. This model was created from a synthesis of a dozen models of human development, my own experience with strength training over the past two decades as well as watching the various communities of individuals practicing strength training around me. The following stage model offers you one particular path through which you may see your own training transform[16].

As you will see, with each stage an emergent novelty expands your faculties, thus liberating you from previous limitations. The practice of your strength training as well as your self system becomes more integrative, thereby enabling you to manage and negotiate greater complexity and more territory of yourself, your training and ultimately your life. These creative emergences manifest in direct response to the inherent limitations of their preceding stages. This understanding of the creative emergence and the evolution of strength training will set an important framework for Part Three of our exploration of engagement and the beacon of performance in your practice. But first let us explore the proposed developmental stages of strength training.

The Path to Mastery

Within the following proposed framework, strength training unfolds in five major stages of development, culminating in Mastery. Stage one, the Building stage, is where you learn the basic dos and don'ts regarding proper breathing techniques and form within any given training modality used to elicit specific physiological responses. Examples of these would be to exhale on the contraction phase of a lift, and properly using various forms that are used to either isolate or integrate muscle groups, increase movement efficiency and/or protect your joints.

Individuals training within this stage are limited by their neuromuscular system's ability to coordinate and integrate new movement patterns and their psychological capacity to remain focused. Focus is often fragmented. For example, attention focuses on lengthening the exhalation through the concentric range of movement during a lunge. As focus is consumed by breathing properly, the form of keeping the knees in line with the feet is lost. As focus shifts back to the proper neurological recruitment of the legs, the individual begins to hold his breath again. Attention then may jump to another dimension regarding the form before being distracted in frustration. This is a common pattern for this stage where integrated neuromuscular coordination requires persistent effort, as attention jumps from one part of the basics to another, form begins to break down. Diligence is required for the neuromuscular foundations of training to be established.

Stage two, the Achieving stage, is where you have gained an adequate level of competence over the basic forms of a particular approach (or perhaps several approaches) to strength training. Neuromuscular foundations have been appropriately established such that breath and form can be efficiently and effectively integrated within a single field of focus. This larger field of focus demonstrates greater integrative capacity. And therefore the focus of training often takes on a new texture at this stage. The basics, no longer requiring heightened effort or feeling foreign and or awkward, are competently employed to achieve an end.

Achievers, or individuals training in this second stage, are by definition training to accomplish a goal. For example, within your strength training you may want to set an objective to increase your power output by 10 percent, or lose an inch off your waistline. Strength training in this modality starts to gain in intensity as it is now purposeful and driven toward a specific goal. Training is not defined by the fundamentals. Instead the Achiever has transcended the fundamentals and included them in an overarching aim. The novel teleological ingredient is evident throughout their training. As such, neuromuscular capacity and psychological focus increase and the result is an entirely new stage of training. While results are pursued with vigor, this stage is limited by the division between body and mind. In the Achieving stage practitioners are identified with their aim and goals in their mind, which seeks to move their body. The mind "rides upon" the body, often struggling to achieve a certain level of obedience with the body.

These two stages of strength training are the predominant forms enacted by the trainers around the world today. The majority of people will get only the occasional glimpse beyond these two stages because these are the stages that are most overtly related to the general functioning of the ego.

If your ego is in command chances are that you are enacting one of these two stages.

The third stage is the Growing stage. While this stage is still egoically governed, the ego's ability to embrace takes a qualitative leap into greater integrative capacity. The defining feature of this stage is an integrated body-mind. Individuals training in this stage have transcended the inherent limitations of identifying with a mind that has a body. They are identified with a self that is larger and more capable when compared to their less mature self, which divides body and mind, thereby splitting physical and mental resources.

As mental, emotional and physical capacities grow and become more integrated, training inhabits a new landscape. First, intention is no longer largely confined to future-oriented goals. Intention now is able to turn to the present moment in which the sole aim is to become unified or integrated into the precise movements of strength training. The experience is first one of *growing* into the present moment, thus the title of this stage. As this body-mind integration refines, this "flow[17]" state, which is an enjoyable and, at times, ecstatic experience, commands intention, attention and engagement in training.

Future-oriented goals still remain, as they are included in the more integrative scope and functioning found in this stage of training. The conventional results of increased strength, flexibility and other more traditional benefits become more and more a welcomed byproduct, but no longer hold the sole purpose and core meaning of why the individual engages in strength training. Getting into this enjoyable training state creates a novel purpose that draws the practitioner into their training day in and day out, repetition after repetition, and breath by breath.

The integrated body-mind's novel capacities allow for the efficient management of attention, thoughts and imagery. As the sense of self has been liberated from an exclusive identification with mind, mental faculties become tools to be leveraged in training. With the newfound integration of the body, emotional and physical energy are conducted through the training movements with greater will, precision and purpose. The result is a more engaged strength training experience with an expanded capacity for precision in the execution of training.

As an added benefit this focus upon engaging the present moment coupled with the self's novel developmental emergences improves performance and consequently delivers conventional results more quickly and easily. Often it is the dogged pursuit for performance that challenges the body and mind to go beyond conventions that set the foundation for this stage of strength training. As experienced practitioners will attest, the highest levels of performance are most often attained in the complete cessation of seeking future aims. It is here that we find the body and moving as one.

The fourth stage of strength training is the Thriving stage. It is defined by the presence of the genuine expressions of passion and inspiration. Here the activity of strength training becomes a passionately driven and inspired activity. While the terms "passion" and "inspiration" are used quite often, these terms are specifically pointing to a part of the self that is beyond the ego. By definition, as these terms are being used here, passion and inspiration are something that cannot be held, managed nor created by your ego. No amount of managing thoughts, imagery, emotions and so on will connect you with your passion and inspiration. Your ego simply cannot generate these phenomenon in their true essence.

Thriving's developmental progression necessitates a liberation from the confines and limitations of ego. No longer is the activity of strength training governed by habituated struggle. Training now supersedes the limited attachment to and investment in enjoyable flow-like experiences. As a result, strength training's deeper core begins to show itself. Training is discovered to be a natural out-movement of one's passion and inspiration for living life fully.

Thriving embodies complete trust in the present moment and one's capacity to experience this fullness with integrity. Where the Growing stage actively focuses *on* the moment, to genuinely thrive you must *be* the moment's expression as you. This is an unmediated aliveness. Experience here is often intense in that your body-mind participates with your direct embodied experience without the layers of egoic struggle. Passion and inspiration open your body-mind to deep levels of joy and pain. When pain is present, living life fully is experiencing pain in a raw, direct, open and unguarded way. When pleasure is present, living fully is inhabiting and embracing the totality of this pleasure without constraint.

Living life fully is experienced as intrinsically joyful. The novel congruence your body-mind inhabits with and as the moment enables you to experience a joy that reaches beyond both pain and pleasure. There is a texture of joyfulness in this transcendence yet also a complete embrace of both pain and pleasure. Fundamentally this joyfulness that integrates and unifies the polarity of pain and pleasure is aliveness itself.

Passion and inspiration are initially attractive concepts for the ego, and it appears, at least at first, that ego may be attempting to create a relationship with these powerful forces within its search for happiness. At a more root level (and thus, in an often unconscious fashion) your ego will be resisting passion and inspiration. The precise activity of egoic struggle in the moment is a resistance to the unmediated aliveness of your already present experience. This unmediated aliveness is the singular source for genuine passion and inspiration, and as such, training within the Thriving stage resides beyond the ego's control.

Taking control away from your ego and allowing passion and inspiration to genuinely guide your training challenges your ego's fundamental stance toward the present moment. Put bluntly, your ego cannot run the show anymore. Its autonomy is negated by the emerging causative agents we are calling passion and inspiration. As a result, this stage of strength training requires a deconstruction of the various strategies your habituation uses to get you from your unmediated experience of the present moment into what you want (consciously or unconsciously) your training experience to be. Put another way, the aliveness that you are beyond your egoic manipulations and contortions is so vibrantly alive that you must literally face death in order to experience it in any consistent fashion.

The deconstruction, dismantling and pulling apart of your ego's habituation is often experienced as an "ego death" of sorts. The price of admission to this stage of training is the complete sacrifice of oneself into the present moment. The identification with the egoic controlling center must come to an end. You have to develop the confidence to "die" into the moment, and as a result, you will gain greater vitality within each moment. Passion and inspiration will burn your habituated ego as this aligned force disassembles much of the ego's conditioned patterns. It is this greater influx of life and vitality into your body-mind from which passion and inspiration genuinely emerge and flower into a guiding intelligence and identity.

Training from this space is what it means to genuinely thrive. Here in this stage the self's managed and guided faculties are not in service of some external future-oriented goal (as in the Achieving stage) nor is it invested in creating an enjoyable experience by entering a flow state (as in the Growing stage) but rather the faculties of self are aligned with the direct immediacy of the heart's passion and inspiration. It is to this aim that all is directed in the unmediated participation with embodied experience.

The fifth and highest proposed stage of strength training is Mastery. It is here in Mastery that we find the ultimate source of your Excellence as we have discussed earlier. For the first time in an embodied full understanding, strength trainers are able to integrate the immense importance of Surrender within their strength training. This Surrender is a movement *into* in addition to *being* your greatest liberation. No longer are you confined to a body-mind doing strength training. Mastery entails knowing in the practitioner's direct, unmediated experience their unbounded infinity. As the eternal changeless liberation, the master inhabits, embraces and enacts her body-mind's unique gifts and talents. Mastery is the source of Excellence.

The previous stage is limited through its investment in the activity of deconstructing habituation in service of the experience and enactment of passion and inspiration. The master's liberation reaches beyond the split between habituation and liberation and experiences these as no longer two separate dimensions of experience. As such, Mastery is characterized by a progressive and rigorous reconstruction of habituation that aligns with and serves not unconscious struggle but a radical embodiment of love in training (and life). No longer is training an attempt to disidentify from habituated activity into purer and purer passion and inspiration. Rather this stage of training actively participates in the construction of Excellence's greatest integrity in the moment. Liberated habituation in service of Excellence is the essence of this stage.

Strength training is allowed to be a complete vehicle for the refinement of Excellence. It is experienced as the natural eventuality of form taking shape in ever-refined constructions of elegant love. Mastery is the culmination of a timeless integration of discipline and play, pain and pleasure, habituation and liberation, as well as effort and Surrender. It is the union or yoga of the One and the Many, Being and Becoming, Form and Formless, and the ascent into transcendence with the descent into immanent embodiment. Mastery is the culmination of who you genuinely are[18], and it is within this space that the master enacts everything from the sacred to the mundane, with weights in hand.

Through discipline and your intention's proper orientation the process of strength training is allowed to flourish and carry you forward into the larger Excellence your life, training, performance and development require of you. Leave out discipline and your clear intention and you risk remaining locked in a constant moment-to-moment struggle governed by your habituated ego. Fail to enact this path and your Excellence dissolves as your training, life and sense of self is governed by a fragment of your genuine possibility. Fail to pick up the path beyond, and you will not transform. Rather, you will entrench your conditioning as life slips by, skimming only a surface of your divine calling to live without habituated reservation.

As you will see in your own practice, the intention to engage wholeheartedly is often in and of itself a novel emergence providing direction and guidance beyond your habituated ego. The presence of this guiding orientation also allows for more space for other dimensions of yourself to emerge with greater ease, elegance and higher proficiency. As engaging wholeheartedly is joined together with your discipline, your commitment to train day in and day out, year in and year out, you have a powerful foundation to evolve through strength training's major stages. The stability of your discipline provides a powerful vehicle through which the novel emergences of your ongoing growth and development can flourish and your Excellence can continually excel beyond previous limitations. With intention and discipline properly aligned you have a potent formula for growth and transformation beyond the conventional norms of your ego's habits and conditioning.

Chapter Eleven
Body-Mind-Moment Training

Thus far we have been establishing the foundations for a new training methodology that can liberate strength training from its conventions and, more importantly, liberate you from the limitations of your ego's habituation. The Integral Practice that we have been carving out is called Body-Mind-Moment Training (BMT). This training methodology transforms you from an egoic mental identity to an integrated body-mind where body and mind are unified in a congruent participation with each other. This synthesis of body and mind is only the first step. Next the body-mind is continually yoked into a conscious engagement with the present moment. This union of body, mind and moment is the central aim.

This methodology integrates, aligns and engages your major faculties into the present moment. Through each movement of strength training, BMT catalyses a synthesis of many of your major capacities and their creative expressions. This integrative training framework is capable of fostering and elevating the articulation of your Excellence. This approach to training expands your access to, and recognition of, your greatest liberation while also growing and refining the unique gifts, skills and talents intrinsic to your Excellence.

This approach can spark your development on the path to mastery regardless of where you may be in your strength training. BMT is a strong foundation for you whether you are learning the fundamentals of strength training, working to enhance your strength, power or other performance metrics, applying yourself to reshaping and re-sculpting your physique or focusing on increasing and refining your capacities on the more subtle and nuanced parts of yourself that lead up to mastery.

This integrated approach is anchored in a framework that is beyond ego. As a result, BMT offers a constant stimulus to train beyond the more conventional approaches to strength training by enacting practices that promote ongoing multifaceted growth. These basic principles and processes are designed to continually pull you into a wakeful and alive engagement with your training, thus actualizing and moving you toward embodying and articulating your greater potential.

One of the basic guiding principles is engaging wholeheartedly. To engage wholeheartedly is neither purely a mental act nor simply a physical act, but requires the integration of your body and mind in the moment. We will investigate your engagement as it pertains to BMT in Section Three; however, for now, please note that as a result of BMT's multidimensional engagement, you yield multidimensional benefits naturally and in some cases effortlessly.

The body in Body-Mind-Moment Training represents both the physical and emotional faculties. BMT therefore refines a number of different lines of development within both of these dimensions. For example, your body can grow in strength and power at an accelerated rate with BMT as can your kinesthetic intelligence, flexibility and aerobic capacity. Emotionally, strength training often is effective at combating depression[19] in addition to positively impacting general affect and mood[20]. BMT also supports the development of critical "self authoring[21]" emotional faculties not characteristic in more conventional approaches to strength training. BMT actively develops highly useful skills to both manage and generate useful emotional states while training. As you will learn through practice, BMT teaches you how to effectively take more responsibility for your emotions, manage the full spectrum of feelings as well as generate positive emotional states on demand to facilitate high levels of execution in your training. As a result, BMT impacts your overall emotional intelligence just as much as it improves your physical strength, immune system, bone density and so on.

Mind is referring to your mental and spiritual faculties. Naturally the multidimensional benefits are not exclusive to just your body as we have been discussing it. BMT also uniquely impacts your mental and spiritual faculties. While findings support strength training's ability to improve the executive functioning of the brain after training sessions[22], BMT unlocks a more important benefit as it fundamentally shifts your self sense to an awareness that is trans-discursive, meaning beyond the linear thinking mind. As a result, discursive thinking can be more easily observed and thus leveraged as a tool for engagement rather than a compulsion for egoic identity.

For example, BMT helps individuals see their conventional egoic thought patterns as they arise during training. This facilitates the growth process through its differentiation phase[23]. Equally important though, as the discursive faculty becomes less and less a vehicle for self identification, it is able to be leveraged as a tool to facilitate engaging more fully into the process of strength training.

As you invest less and less of your energy into your habituated discursive story lines, your mental flexibility increases, enabling your cognitive faculties to be devoted to refining and guiding your engagement. Additionally your liberated cognitive faculties are able to animate your guiding intention with more force, track various types of goals, and engage in forms of self-talk that can facilitate an ever-evolving approach to your training.

Another important part of the cognitive faculty is visualization. For example, visualization can be leveraged to mentally and emotionally rehearse for your training. You may also learn how to use visualization before each set to unlock a greater degree of engagement and refined execution throughout each exercise as you approach higher and higher levels of intensity, performance and execution in your training.

As your BMT matures and you begin to master your body-mind's engagement with the moment you will start to leverage trans-verbal imagery (imagery that transcends the linear discursive cognitive framework as a whole). This form of imagery involves highly integrative images that communicate intention, a sense of identity and tremendous amounts of multilayered information, and these images do this all in the immediacy of the moment. Vast amounts of information are integrated into these images, such as form, posture, mood, emotional quality, intensity, mental focus, attentional placement and so on. Your body-mind will naturally integrate this critical faculty of imagery and develop it in BMT's approach to engagement and the execution of your strength training.

Your spiritual faculties are impacted by integrating meditative and contemplative practices into the practice of strength training. As we briefly touched on in chapter nine, contemplation refers to an inquiry into yourself and your training, while meditation refers to practices that animate your trans-egoic witnessing faculties as well as your ability to connect with your most basic way of Being.

To give another example, BMT refines your ability for inquiry through its reflective mechanism built into its program structure. While there is a period of reflection set aside after your training, BMT is also designed for you to confront your ego and some of the most basic existential questions: Who am I? What is my will? What originates my movement? What experiences this moment? and so on. These are all questions that emerge spontaneously and increasingly begin to frustrate[24] your identification to your conventional sense of self. As a result, your ability to be consumed by serious inquiry will naturally refine.

Equally important, BMT also cultivates your capacity for meditation. As you learn to engage your highest levels of refined execution you will find stillness within the immense power and movement flowing through your body-mind. This stillness is the root of and foundation for all meditation. Similarly, as your capacity to Surrender and recover between sets improves, you will learn how to consciously rest in this essential seat of Being (your ever-present wakefulness as the unmoved mover, the non-seeking stillness.) Mastering meditation within strength training is one of the central benefits from the cultivation of mastery within this rich discipline.

The Here and Now

A common assumption many people hold is that being fully in the present is "not thinking." This assumption places the ego in a perfect position to struggle with all thought. This egoic stance of eradicating thinking is fundamentally not the trans-egoic relationship with the present moment we are aiming to cultivate in BMT. Thought, as everything else, arises in the moment and is to be intimately engaged with and held by your unconditioned presence, not avoided or eliminated.

Similarly many people impose the assumption that being "in the moment" needs to be peaceful, fulfilling, meaningful, and so on. Again this is your ego's attempt to control what is fundamentally not controllable. All of your assumptions and expectations of being connected and engaged with the here and now are an attempt to manipulate the here and now into something else. This fundamentally misses the territory that is present in the here and now, which includes, at times, your ego's attempt to control and manipulate. Sometimes your training experience will be more peaceful and fulfilling than anything else you have experienced in life. Other times your training will be mundane and simple. The point here is that you engage with the full unbounded spectrum of all that is arising, without condition, repetition after repetition and set after set.

The present moment is the prime integrator, thus it excludes nothing. As you grow into this moment, you will come to know yourself as the prime integrator, meaning you—the heart of you—will leave nothing out of your embrace of this and every moment. You honor all and allow all to manifest.

BMT is a process to gain greater clarity, from which you can increasingly see your ego's continual attempts to make the here and now into something else. While BMT grows your faculties in a number of different ways, including your ability to witness the subtleties of your ego, fundamentally it is a process of recognizing what you already are, always have been and always will be.

Cultivating a post-conventional relationship with the present moment is based on two basic guiding principles: Accepting and Inhabiting. Accepting is, at its root, not struggling with what is, while Inhabiting involves an intimate engagement with what is. This foundation of Accepting and Inhabitation is not at odds with your ego's struggle.

Acceptance has one fundamental perspective: Receive what is. This receptive faculty is your witness. Acceptance is "taking in" what is. It is the drive to simply witness, that is, to observe, what is.[25] Complimenting Acceptance is Inhabitation, which involves an active "moving out" into manifestation as manifestation. The drive to engage, relate and be seen are all aspects of Inhabiting.[26]

During strength training, Acceptance is exhibited as an unwavering witnessing of what is. It is a presence shining through your open body-mind to receive, take in and witness the present moment without limitation. The scope from which you will witness and accept will vary throughout training; however, the ever-present stance of being vividly aware of what is will not, as your strength training matures. For example, during a set of squats your witnessing capacity will be focused on watching your particular body-mind's posture, breath and the quality of engagement as your set of squats progresses. After this set, the witnessing stance may broaden to take in a larger field of manifestation. For example you may notice the sunlight on a wall, other people in the gym and the felt space of the entire gym. Your witnessing field may become ever more flexible so as to shift from a laser-like focus to one of a broader more expansive stance.

During this same set your active Inhabitation is the actual force of the intention and drive animating your body-mind. This is the active effort that focuses your mind, channels your emotional energy and engages your muscular system throughout your squats. When you cultivate this post-conventional relationship with the present moment based on Acceptance and Inhabitation, you can integrate the two core drives to witnessing manifestation and enacting the basic movement of manifestation through your training.

A wide spectrum of benefits emerges from this high-level integration as your BMT evolves. Among them is your vivid experience of a larger expanse from which all of yourself and ultimately all of manifestation emerges. As your relationship with this field evolves you will learn to animate and channel this larger field of vitality throughout your body-mind. This spaciousness is simply the larger field of the here and now to which you are intimately connected. Cultivating a conscious connection with this seat of Being and learning how to act from this authentic seat of strength stands at the core of developing your meditative faculties and is one of the core dimensions of your Excellence, and thus stands as a central aim of BMT.

Training

Training refers to a purposeful, disciplined and intentional engagement with the moment. BMT is purposeful both in its conventional sense of obtaining a wide spectrum of typical outcome goals as well as executing on key process goals necessary for engaging the true aim of strength training. To give an example of how BMT leverages both conventional and post-conventional goals, let us consider some of the following end results you may desire to achieve through BMT. You may want to lose weight, preserve or increase lean muscle tissue, improve strength metrics, increase your capacity for power output, improve your capacity for progressive acceleration, refine your performance capacities for a sport, promote your psychological well-being, refine your executive functioning, cultivate your spiritual awareness away from your meditation cushion and so on. These are all useful purpose-driven goals that provide meaning to your training. These goals provide a valid answer to the question: Why do you strength train?

While answering the question "Why?" is foundational, you cannot stop there. That is why BMT drives beyond these conventional goals in its focus on what is referred to as process goals. Process goals focus solely on this one question: How?

How are you going to achieve this desired end? How are you going to get from here to there? Process goals provide the moment-to-moment cues to follow and execute on leading you in the proper direction. To give an example, the process of generating the quickest, most explosive movements with perfect form focuses the mind and energy into proper alignment and expression necessary to develop athletic power. Each repetition has a process that is to be followed providing structure and guidance to ensure more efficient and effective training adaptations. Another process goal that might be coupled with this training methodology is to stop the set as soon as the fastest range of motion is lost. This dictates when you stop as to again ensure training is focusing upon refining explosive power and not other training outcomes. Yet another process goal could be to produce the most amount of power with the least amount of effort. This process goal helps negotiate a certain level of qualitative engagement with the present moment that refines your capacity to perform or articulate your peak levels of execution as you are training.

Process goals are centrally important for BMT because they do not focus on outcomes. Outcome goals are always projections into the future. Instead, process goals focus on themselves and directly connect with what is going on in the present moment. When skillfully crafted and properly chosen, process goals accelerate your results by evolving your moment-to-moment engagement with your training and the critical and most relevant processes to focus on and refine. As a result, these goals provide a powerful bridge to the transcendent dimensions of strength training ,which you will learn more about in Part Three.

Training in BMT is disciplined in that it provides the boundaries and structure to shift beyond your conventional sense of self and typical ways of being and functioning in your training. BMT provides a source of delight, energy and, ultimately, freedom from your ego's entrapment. BMT elicits the unconditional choice to fully engage with this rich Integral Practice.

Finally, BMT is intentional as it is built from your intention upward. Intention ultimately dictates where you end up, and as a result, this unique form of training specifically cultivates your ability to set and maintain a strong connection with your core driving intention(s) in your strength training. This form of training stands as the freedom from conventional forms of exercise.

Let us now turn our attention to the heart of Body-Mind-Moment Training and how the beacon of human performance calls out to your emerging Excellence.

Part Three:
The Art of Engagement &
The Beacon of Performance

Sometimes the culmination of the practice
manifests as I simply set up the weights for
another person. As I glance into his eyes, he
says thank you, and his gratitude washes
through me and breaks open my heart. I am
shocked into tears as I walk to my next
exercise. I think to myself, "Kindness ...
kindness ... kindness" with long drafts of
spaciousness surrounding everything. I
remind myself, "These simple acts are the
heart of true strength."

Chapter Twelve

Engagement: The Heart of Body-Mind-Moment Training

> At some point I stopped trying to find the right
> posture. Suddenly, seemingly out of nowhere, I
> ceased my conventional approaches to form and
> posture. Something new emerged in my practice
> as the right posture, the precise posture my
> body-mind ached for, found me. In this subtle
> inner movement everything changed; I was the
> moving embodiment of Stillness. I felt as if all of
> my searching culminated in this release, and
> suddenly my capacity to perform flowered into
> something I was not able to possess, yet
> miraculously was articulating right here and
> right now as me in this moment.

At the heart of Body-Mind-Moment Training we find the practice of engagement, or "engaging wholeheartedly." The role of intention helps establish a live connection with your training and practice as opposed to an unconscious habituated relationship to training. This sets the foundation from which your engagement rests. As explored in Chapter Eight, the role of engaging wholeheartedly is central. Discipline then provides the framework, structure and boundaries for your training to unfold. Fragment yourself from engaging in your training, fail to cut a live intention, fail to establish and Surrender into a discipline that holds the entirety of your training and practice, and you can no longer consider your strength training BMT.

While intention and discipline are critically important elements, the heart of BMT is engaging wholeheartedly. Part of engaging wholeheartedly includes acknowledging the intention to create and allow a new relationship with the present moment to emerge. This intention has two essential parts. The first is that by opening ourselves to something new, by allowing a space for novelty to emerge in its fullness we are asking ourselves to set aside projects to try to re-create an experience we have had in the past. This most overtly takes the shape of trying to recreate a particularly good or enjoyable training session. Engaging wholeheartedly is not, at its heart, about creating what was or replaying the past but rather with connecting more completely with what is right now in this vibrant moment. This may indeed be something similar to what we have encountered in the past, however we are allowing ourselves to embody a liberated spaciousness to hold much more in our training. With BMT you are creating an attuned connection with the present moment.

The second part of the intention to engage wholeheartedly is to ask yourself to put aside projects in order to create a fantasy or idealistic experience that you think you should have. Just like we are not trying to recreate a past experience, we are not trying to impose an expectation or set of expectations about how your training experience should be. Together these two sides—the willingness to not recreate past experiences and the willingness to not manufacture expectations—establish the essential foundation from which a novel relationship to the present moment can unfold. Once you have established this larger framework, once you have embodied and integrated this stance toward the present moment, you will embrace a greater curiosity toward and animate your training from a larger spaciousness. You will enact your training from a part of you that is fundamentally unconditioned. It is from this starting point that BMT holds six major stages [27] of engagement.

The Six Stages of Engagement

These six stages begin with the most basic and fundamental instructions and articulate a particular way of engaging with your training. As you ascend to subsequent stages the more refined and advanced the instruction becomes and the more depth of engagement your training will embody. This spectrum of engagement is a holarchy in that each stage stands as a whole and distinct level of engagement and each stage's functional attributes are embraced and integrated into the next stage of engagement. Thus as your training develops over time you will continue to embrace the most basic and fundamental forms of engagement as your training continues to evolve. In this process of refinement you do not only transcend, but also include. You go beyond and also integrate. Your training supersedes yet simultaneously embraces the essential functions of all preceding stages of engagement.

Stage 1: Breath—Conducting Energy

Breathing is the foundation of engagement in BMT. Resting your attention on the breath as you synchronize your breathing to each movement is the first stage. Generally speaking, breath is expelled during the concentric phase of each movement. The concentric phase of movement involves a concentric muscular contraction in which the working muscles shorten, thus generating force. The breath can be either forcefully and rapidly expelled or slowly but powerfully expelled during the contraction of the major muscle groups being trained (depending on the type of training being performed.) Breath is then taken in during the negative eccentric phase of each movement. In this phase an eccentric extension elongates the working muscle. Again, breathing may vary from a rapid inhalation to a slow and controlled inhalation based on the specific training modality being used.

For example, you would exhale as you stand up out of a chair while your major leg muscles contract, lifting your body from a seated position into a standing position. As you lower your body back down into the chair you would then inhale during this eccentric contraction of your leg muscles. Similarly you would exhale as you push yourself up from the ground during a pushup as your triceps and chest muscles concentrically contract, and then inhale as you lower yourself eccentrically back to the ground. This is the most basic foundation of the rhythm between breath and movement.

There are exceptions to this basic rhythm as there are exercises in which the body-mind's ability for greater engagement and higher levels of intensity can be animated when cyclical breathing patterns are integrated. For example, as high levels of intensity are achieved you may spontaneously begin to cycle breath in and out rapidly as a single movement is performed to conduct greater energy through the body-mind. Another exception is when the basic exhale/inhale integration with concentric/eccentric contractions are reversed. In some movements additional stability in the chest and shoulders during the contraction phase of a movement is useful. You may respond to these demands by reversing the basic breathing pattern by then inhaling during the contraction phase and exhaling during the eccentric lowering phase of each movement.

Another important dimension to this stage of engagement is attending to the type of breath. For our purposes we will focus on two basic types of breathing: thoracic and diaphragmatic. Thoracic breathing involves inhaling into the chest and ribcage without dropping the air down into the belly and releasing the abdominal muscles. Thoracic breathing is used most frequently during each set of an exercise as this most readily integrates with your nervous system as it manages high levels of stress and physical intensity.

In between sets you will learn to employ diaphragmatic breathing. Diaphragmatic breathing is associated with physiological and psychological states of relaxation and a greater transport of oxygen in the lungs. Your nervous system relaxes, and your body-mind absorbs energy with greater efficiency when diaphragmatic breathing patterns are adopted. Following the completion of a set your breath will begin transitioning from breathing powerfully into the chest toward breathing downward allowing the breath to fill and extend the belly.

Some diaphragmatic breathing will be integrated into your sets, specifically for adding stability to your lower spine while performing leg based exercises; the difference here will be that your abdominal muscles will retain high degrees of tension as you breathe down into your belly, thus adding stability to your core and subsequently your lower spine. Diaphragmatic breathing between sets is different in that the abdominal muscles are released and relaxed as the breath drops thus extending the belly outward.

Many people have an unconscious relationship with how they breathe and the various types of breath they have available to them. As a result many months can be spent solely focused on learning the various ways the body-mind relates to breath and how these breathing patterns intersect with various exercises. If BMT is engaged properly, breathing continues to be a learning platform and is never in its entirety learned or mastered. Practitioners should expect to go through periods of pronounced work on the intentional use of breath in which these patterns and forms of breathing are learned and integrated into their body-mind's repertoire. Intentional shifts in focus or at times spontaneous shifts in engagement may then move the practitioner's overall stage of engagement with their training. Often novel breathing patterns and strategies emerge as engagement develops and refines, thus continually integrating this ever-present source of engagement. Regardless of how you train, the foundation for engagement remains in the wedding of your attention to the breath as you move through your training, both while you execute your exercises and while you recover between each set.

Stage 2: Form—Animating the Posture

Form is the second stage of engagement. It is the movement of your body-mind through specific ranges of motion sequenced together. Form is most commonly taught through demonstration and a set of positive and negative injunctions relating to posture, alignment and technique. For example, while doing Shoulder Lateral Raises with dumbbells the following might unfold while learning form. I would demonstrate posture and technique with specific instructions:

Your knees are slightly bent. Do not lock out your knees at any point during this exercise. Maintain a slight bend in the elbows. Hold this angle in the elbow joints throughout the exercise, both on the way up and the way down. Your palms remain facing the ground at the top of this movement. Explode powerfully at the bottom of the movement when the weights are close to your sides. Continue a steady strong cadence until your hands are parallel with your shoulders. Pause briefly.

Proper form as understood and practiced in BMT is articulated through the joining of body and mind into precise movements and expressions of each exercise performed. While you may contain perfect form from an objective standpoint, your mind must be directly in connection with the movement itself. You cannot simply ingrain a habitual physical form and then allow your mind to wander.

Beginners often start out with a greater attentiveness to the details of their movements as they learn new exercises. However, stage two intermediate practitioners commonly fall into the trap of divorcing the body and mind from one another once they assume they have learned and understood the proper form of a movement. This is a major hindrance to the cultivation of more refined stages of engagement, which we will discuss shortly. However, for many people their path through this stage of engagement is that of a "U."

The beginner starts off focused, attentive and curious as to how to perform an exercise properly. They correctly focus their mind on learning the various parts of the movement, yet often incorrectly assume proper form just involves the body. As their training progresses in terms of the neural and muscular integration of each exercise, their mind often becomes more and more disengaged. Daydreaming and the wandering of attention are perhaps the most common of these pitfalls. As the practitioner begins to mature, form begins to be understood as the exquisitely refined movement of the body with one's mental focus and attention wedded to each movement. It is through this maturation that the third stage of engagement begins to transition and give rise to the next stage of engagement.

Stage 3: Sensation—Riding Immediacy

The Sensation stage of engagement is characterized by the alive union of body and mind found in the direct immediacy of felt experience. This stage enacts a refined attunement with the moment-to-moment embodied experience of training. When breath and form have been integrated sufficiently this new attunement emerges with the movements of training. Your intimacy with direct sensations rests in your ever-refining awareness and embodiment of both breath and form. Your attention closely follows and inhabits the movements of the body-mind by directly entering into the embodied sensations of training.

As your practice evolves over time, attention is no longer directed with effort in order to follow your training movements as an observing faculty (marking a mature stage 2 engagement). With sufficient and properly directed practice your body-mind's focused presence continues to strengthen and dive further into engaging the moment. This results in your mind ceasing to observe your movements from the outside where consciousness begins to intimately feel and embody the movements from the inside of sensation. Form conventionally holds a more prescriptive or controlling relationship to the movement where the mind imposes or enforces strategies and methodologies upon the body. This third stage of engagement embodies a novel ingredient: the letting go of an exclusively prescriptive relationship with your body-mind. Instead of your mind watching breath and form from the outside and directing your training your attention dives directly into the embodied immediacy of the movement. Here the conventional, or directing, volitional faculty is released. As this directing faculty is let go, a more integrated body-mind embracing greater spontaneity and attunement with the present moment emerges.

This new volitional faculty does not belong to the conventional self's habituation. Control is released into a participation with the spontaneous unfolding of the body-mind's activity. Sometimes this movement is characterized by an expansion of energy, increased fluidity of awareness and greater conductivity of power through the graceful participation with what is most alive. Other times the spontaneous expression will be that of engaging sensations of closing down and working with that which is frozen, stuck and collapsed within your body-mind.

While a novice observer may not see differences in form as they watch someone training from this stage of engagement, the practitioner training from sensation experiences each repetition, breath and movement as a unique aliveness where each subtlety is fundamentally precious and infinitely captivating. This aliveness is due in large part to the releasing of control of the conditioned directing volitional faculty. What results is an intimate embrace of the heat, vibration, texture and flow of sensation throughout the body-mind and the spontaneous emergence of your body-mind's natural intelligence of the conductivity and articulation of energy.

Within this stage there is an open curiosity within the body-mind's exploration of form and breath. As sensation is explored and inhabited through your training, attention and energy flow together as one throughout the body-mind from your toes to your crown. Training that emphasizes pushing resistance away and extending energy out into the world conducts consciousness and energy up from your feet and legs up along your spine through an open heart and out the arms. As you press outward and extend with grace, your spine lengthens and the crown of your head floats away from your shoulders. Your breath and form naturally follow that which is most alive in the moment. Training that emphasizes drawing resistance toward your spine, powerfully enlivening the muscles of your back, conducts energy from your fingertips down the arms into a flowering open heart that radiates fluid energy up and down the spine.

Training from this third stage retains the alignment and technique learned from stage 2 and the ability to conduct energy fluidly with breath. Breath and form, however, are only a structure or framework within which the body-mind dives into and enacts. Subtle spontaneous shifts in posture, alignment, technique and/or breath are explored as each movement unfolds uniquely. It is this attunement with the direct immediacy of sensation that marks this third stage of engagement within BMT.

The Leap

It is often through considerable practice at stage three that the next stage begins to emerge in any consistent fashion. This is not to diminish the importance of stage-four states that temporarily open your eyes to a new way of being and functioning in your training (and the world at large) while you are primarily working on the fundamentals of engagement. These temporary glimpses of "the beyond" often facilitate the evolution of your training.

By refining your engagement into sensation you will at some point spontaneously make what I call *The Leap*. Prior to The Leap you will experience yourself as a body-mind that is doing the training. You will feel yourself as a dynamically attuned body-mind animating your training in the moment. This is the "you" before The Leap. After The Leap, you will experience yourself as a stillness within which your body-mind moves. This new seat of awareness transcends your habituated attachment to your body-mind's perception. The novel stillness that emerges after The Leap is the boundless spaciousness of the unconditioned presence of Being which stretches far beyond your relative body-mind. Your body-mind's breath, form and sensation are held within this expansive stillness. This is the dimension of you that never moves, yet always holds and embraces all movement.

Stage 4: Being—Spaciousness meets Stillness

The forth stage of engagement involves a dramatic shift in subjectivity. Prior to The Leap your subjectivity is tethered to and attached with your body-mind. Afterwards your subjectivity is no longer exclusively identified with your body-mind. Thus your faculty of perception is no longer limited to only your relative body-mind. Your perceptual faculties drop through, or leap beyond, your body-mind, expanding to participate with your most essential seat of Being.

When you enter into this fourth stage of engagement you experience the moment from the subjective seat of limitless Being. Your presence and perspective inhabits an incredible depth of stability and equanimity that is unconditioned. This is to say the infinite stillness that is the heart of

Being is not dependent upon anything. Being is fundamentally liberated in its limitless spaciousness. This infinite field of Being is a new level of engagement providing an unqualifiable experience of peace that intrinsically embraces and articulates immense power, strength and grace.

As you are training from Being, stillness pervades all that is arising in the moment without any limitation. Conducting extreme forms of movement through your body-mind has no influence upon the utter depth of Being's unmoving presence. For the first time, practitioners are no longer a body-mind in the moment, rather they are a body-mind arising *as* the moment. The unfolding, changing and evolving nature of their body-mind's Becoming is held within the moment's infinite seat of Being. Body-Mind-Moment Training has taken a monumental leap forward in this shift in perception, which alters the practitioners' capacity to engage their training in novel ways.

For example, while doing a bent-over dumbbell row you may make The Leap beyond your more limited body-mind and suddenly inhabit the infinite expanse of space. You feel your leg grounding into the earth and your hand and knee stabilizing your spine into the bench. Your attention is still flowing within the energy as you draw the dumbbell toward your opening heart, and the back of your heart powerfully draws your arm upwards and your shoulder blades ache together and pull downward along your back as your spine subtly arches forward, pressing your heart into the world with clarity. You feel the crown of your head extend and float away from your tail bone as they extend towards an infinite horizon. As the heat and vibration increase and your body-mind focuses, suddenly The Leap occurs. You are still experiencing all of this unfolding within your limited body-mind, but something dramatic has shifted: You have inhabited your infinite body-mind. Along with the intensity of your training you also feel the inside of limitless stillness. Just as you feel your own muscles conducting consciousness and energy through them, you feel the peaceful expanse and equanimity of unconditioned Being. You feel your limited body-mind struggling with the intensity of your training, yet in this open, unconditioned embrace, all is held in a perfect embrace. Your struggle is inhabited more fully precisely because you are fully liberated from all limitation and conditioning. Training continues to unfold moment after moment with each sliver of movement held and known within the infinite seat of Being.

Being's unconditioned liberation from all Becoming provides practitioners with a groundless ground from which a novel articulation of Excellence unfolds emergent capacities for higher and higher levels of performance. Training your body-mind within this stage enables the conventional body-mind to enact seemingly superhuman feats of strength, endurance, agility and so on. The limitless expanse of Being increases your capacity to go beyond conditioned limitations precisely because you are no longer exclusively identified with those limitations. Any attempt to grasp at, own, possess or in any other way control such emergent faculties severs your engagement from Being and halts the ongoing development of your engagement and training.

Stage 5: Mystery—Awakening to The Condition

As stage five emerges in training your presence will grow from inhabiting the infinite embrace of Being while training to animating your training from the *origin* of Being. This is a subtle yet powerful shift. Training in the limitless space of Being is qualitatively distinct from the activity of your training penetrating *into* the origin of Being. It is through this act in which Mystery is known and embodied.

This stage first begins to show up as an inquiry into the genesis of Being. These questions can take many different forms; for example, "Who is Being?" "What is witnessing?" and "Where does movement start?" are all expressions of Being's inquiry into its source.

These questions are not merely conceptual musings. These inquiries stem not from your relative body-mind but rather from the transcending seat of Being. Infinity itself is curious about itself. As a result, these inquiries emerge, often spontaneously, within your training. It is within the spaciousness of Being, the direct immediacy of sensation, form and breath that you will experience this core inquiry arising as part of your engagement. The Mystery infuses the heart of your witness to the entirety of your training.

While on a conventional level you may know that you are doing squats, that you are on your fourth repetition and are channeling energy up your spine through the crown of the head as you stand up radiantly and powerfully, at the same time you are in awe at what is causing this. Who is in control? What is shaping this energy? How did this shift in posture arrive to open my heart in this unique particular way? Where does this power originate? Who is experiencing this?

The only authentic answer to these inquiries is that of not knowing. As this stage of engagement matures your inquiries stabilize and eventually fall away leaving only the essence of who you are as the starting point for all of training. This is what I call *awakening to the condition*. You are a silent Mystery at your center. Training at this level originates from and embodies the Mystery, the fundamentally unknowable quality of who you are. As a result, this stage embraces a comfortability with not-knowing-ness. Mystery expands on Being's spaciousness, providing more openness and integrative capacity to birth, hold and embody the creative impulses that stem from your unknown center. This is your foundation for your emergent Excellence calling you into both your greatest freedom and your greatest fullness. It is this embodiment that engaging wholeheartedly is pointing at.

Stage 6: Suchness—Non-duality

While BMT's aim is an integrated animation of stages one through five, there is a sixth stage of engagement, which is more accurately defined as both the ground of all stages of engagement, and the summit and principle aim of all the stages. The ground and foundation of all that is arising (breath, form, sensation, Being and Mystery) is nothing other than the suchness of this all-embracing moment. This suchness is also the summit in that it expresses the fundamental liberation from all duality, as duality. Duality or dualism posits that reality is composed of two kinds of things. Subject and object, individual and collective, mind and body, good and bad, Being and Becoming as well as pleasure and pain are all examples of the perceived dual nature of reality. It is this freedom from duality, this radial boundless liberation, that all engagement yearns for. Fundamentally, your strength training is an expression of this core impulse to reach beyond duality, to experience beyond the duality of self and other, interior and exterior, one and many.

Your reaching beyond limitation ultimately leads you to the precipice, but only in the fullest, fiercest and most complete Surrender will you realize your unconditioned suchness (in which the subject that you have assumed to be for so long is shattered into a liberation that is utterly familiar). The objects you once looked at reveal themselves to be the seat of your subjectivity. You look at all that is arising yet simultaneously experience yourself as all that is arising. Subject and object become not-two, they are non-dual. You find yourself, your most essential self, as that which is non-dual. You are not simply one. You are not simple unity. Distinctions still arise as they always have, but you no longer experience yourself as this part and not that part. You are equally the dumbbells in your hands as you are the eyes looking into the mirror. You still feel your body-mind pressing into and extending into resistance, however you also feel the walls from within. All that is arising is fundamentally not-two, non-dual.

BMT is not aimed at the non-dual because it is the non-dual through and through. Aiming at something would only introduce "this and that" and the non-dual is fundamentally "both this *and* that," or said a different way the non-dual is "neither this *nor* that." There is fundamentally nothing you can do to realize this dimension of engagement aside from practice, and more practice. Eventually this simple recognition will grab you, awakening you to the fullness of life.

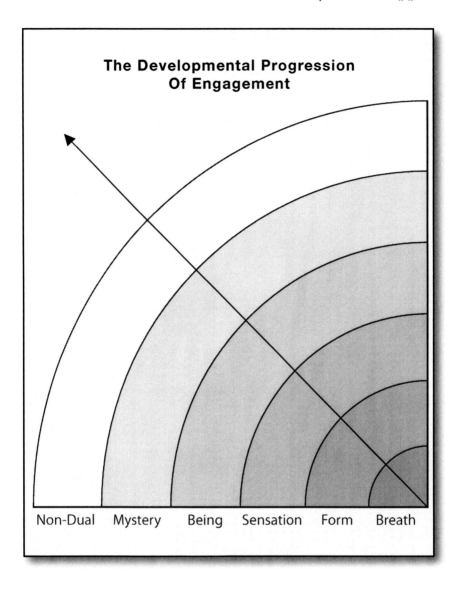

Chapter Thirteen

Resistance: Your Fuel Forward

Engagement's obstacle is resistance. If there is one obstacle impeding the unfolding and development of your Body-Mind-Moment Training it is resistance. As explored in Parts One and Two, the ego's basic process, the moment-to-moment process by which you create and maintain your conventional self, is through a struggle with what is. This habituated and conditioned sense of self, your ego (or conventional self) is resistance through and through. It is this conditioned resistance that takes shape and manifests at each stage of BMT's spectrum of engagement.

In this chapter we will explore the common forms of resistance your conventional sense of self tends to manufacture at each stage of engagement. These are the sticking points that inhibit your training from evolving. However, it is important that you do not attempt to get rid of resistance, as this is just another layer of resistance atop the initial resistance. Furthermore, while resistance is an obstacle to engagement, it is also the incredibly rich means by which you refine your training and engagement.

Resistance is both an obstacle and an indispensable resource to fuel your practice. Whatever resistance makes itself known in the moment is that which is most alive. This is your place to begin working on engagement; this obstacle happening right now is your next step. Some obstacles will crop up overtly and resolve easily, while others will remain hidden for years only to find resolution through heartfelt disciplined practice. Ultimately every resistance is completely unique, a precious opportunity to train, practice and awaken.

That said, let us take a look at some of the typical ways resistance takes shape in each stage of engagement and look at a few techniques and strategies that may be useful as you animate and engage BMT.

Working with Resistance: Habitual Breathing Patterns

Breath is a consistent dynamic presence throughout your training, whether you are just learning to engage the moment through your body-mind or pioneering the depths of the Mystery that is this moment's essence. There is an incredible rich display of breath taking many shapes, textures and tones as you circulate energy throughout your body-mind.

The breath can flow down into the belly. Rebounding off a strongly held core into the sides of the lower back, it can be channeled into the middle back expanding the thoracic spine and rib cage behind the heart. Breath can drop into an open relaxed belly or fill the chest, expanding the rib cage as it stretches and increases your lung capacity. Exhalations can be long and smooth with a cooling, relaxing texture, fast and open, or forceful, channelled and explosive. Your breath can flow up and down your spine in new ways with each breath of air.

The principle aim of breathing is the circulation of energy. Physiologically this means it brings in oxygen and releases respiratory byproducts. Psychologically this is your ever-present anchor to bring your attention and embodied presence into the moment. This is the doorway through which all engagement moves. Your breath is the circulation of your most vital energy source and an open invitation to bring your full awareness into the moment in its full spectrum of expression.

Given the diversity of breath to be explored and animated, one of the biggest obstacles is unconsciously falling into your habitual breathing patterns. We all have at least one habitual breathing pattern. Most of us tend to breathe into the chest for the majority of waking life. Our breathing patterns shift and change rhythmically during sleep as we cycle through dreaming and deep dreamless sleep. However, the majority of us rarely explore the diversity of options through which we can conduct and circulate energy or shift our consciousness and perspective through breath work. Whenever your attention shifts onto your breathing it changes. Similarly, when you forget about your breath entirely or you sever the mind from the body, you typically fall into your habituated way(s) of breathing.

Recall the core intentions that establish the groundwork for BMT's engagement continuum. First, there is the intention to not recreate past experiences, and second there is the intention to not manufacture fantasies or impose expectations upon your training. When you fall into your conditioned breathing patterns, you are often falling into your habituated sense of self, and have lost touch with the two basic intentions that hold the foundation of what it means to engage wholeheartedly with your training. When this happens your habituated self often is governed by the desire to recreate or avoid some experience from the past or get to some preconceived location in the future, neither of which have much depth of a connection with the present moment as it is.

Invariably you will be working with this obstacle. This form of resistance halts you from discovering yourself as an integrated dynamic, body-mind uniquely animated moment to moment. When you notice that you have fallen back into your habitual ways of breathing, that is when you notice that you have been unconscious in your training. Your conditioned self has just been playing out the same old patterns, and you need to go back to square one. Start with the core intentions: 1. Do not attempt to recreate the past and, 2. Do not attempt to manufacture or manipulate the present moment into a fantasy or expectation.

Once you have practiced working with these intentions long enough (and chances are you will spend *many* times at square one) you will be able to connect with them directly and immediately, without having to stop and think them out. With discipline and the proper structure informing your training, you will readily apprehend the critical phrase or core instruction of these intentions. You will be able to recall them and embrace both the awareness of falling back into one's conditioned sense of self, and the aligning of oneself to the critical instructions in BMT's core orienting intentions.

Once you have done the work of connecting and reconnecting, you will be able to catch yourself mid-stride as you fall into your conditioned habitual breathing patterns, and bring yourself right back into connecting with the novelty of each breath as you train.

Working with Resistance: Form's Falling Points

We will treat resistance as it pertains to form in two subsections. The first is oriented to the posture and alignment with the body, and the second is oriented to the posture and alignment of the mind and your attention.

Resistance as Breaks in Physical Posture, Alignment and Technique

Deviation and shifts in the posture and alignment of the body are considered resistance unless they are articulated and embodied by a higher stage of engagement. Thus, if your posture, alignment and movement of an exercise deviates from the prescribed method of movement and is not animated and embodied by sensation, Being, or Mystery, then it is often an unconscious strategy to resist properly training the body-mind.

But what if you learn improper form at the beginning? The sensation stage of engagement provides an important safeguard: The body-mind often adjusts from innate kinesthetic intelligence. You will naturally steer your training toward movements that are better suited to the structural integrity of your body if you are genuinely following BMT and its guiding intentions and practices.

Many problems do stem from being trapped by the conditioned sense of self. Instead of intimately connecting with the body-mind as they train, strength trainers commonly instead ride their body from a place of expectation and try to push it too far, reinforcing a "no pain, no gain" strategy that is often obsessed with attaining an idealistic image or performance expectation.

Whether you have been training for fifteen years largely defined by your conventional self or you have just picked up strength training, the potential for improper form is the same: it is a lack of engagement. The less engaged you are the more potential for breaks in form, and thus the greater potential for injury. In the former, form may be misguided by your conventional sense of self that falls prey to your conditioned history. In the latter, form may be misguided by lack of instruction, a lack of neurological integration, or both.

With that said, your innate kinesthetic intelligence is not going to provide you with all that you need. There is a lot of information that you can learn by studying the human body scientifically that you will never uncover in your first-person exploration of movement with resistance, no matter how engaged you are. These are two different domains of inquiry. Observing the human body from the outside from an objective standpoint illuminates truths that simply cannot be seen and discovered through your own isolated subjective experience; therefore we need to integrate both.

Finding experts in kinesiology, physical therapy, or orthopedic medicine is *absolutely essential* to any serious practitioner. Allow them to educate you on the best way to train, refine movement efficiency, integrate muscle groups, learn how to protect and strengthen joints and so on. You do not necessarily need to get your master's in kinesiology, but the more exposure you have to experts in the field of the human body and how the body moves, the more intelligent your training will become. The sensation stage of engagement is an important safeguard with its attunement to each movement and its subtle nuances, but your overall training intelligence will be multiplied by combining outside expertise with your own innate wisdom.

Resistance has several core expressions here as it pertains to the human body: It is the resistance to learning, adopting and or consistently implementing proper training posture, alignment and technique. Assumptions that modeling others or that your first stab at proper technique is good enough are common expressions of resistance to form. Any general avoidance of expert advice is also a common expression of this type of resistance. However, given different philosophies on movement and the purpose of training, poor technique is contextual.

Given the multiple schools of thought regarding proper form, BMT acknowledges the larger process of learning a diversity of perspectives on form. This starts with a trusted, experienced practitioner or professional. You then adopt and integrate the form as you embrace the instruction in your own practice. It is during this period that you articulate the trust of this particular movement philosophy. At some point in your training you will come across another philosophy of movement, a new way of thinking about how the body is best suited for movement. You may then shift your trust to this instruction and integrate it into your training. A few months or perhaps years later, the same process will happen again. Sometimes you may adopt an entirely new movement philosophy. Other times you will add and integrate only the most important parts for you as you grow and refine your own integrated movement philosophy.

The critical point here is that while there are periods of learning, consolidation and integration, you never fully arrive at *the* single way to perform an exercise and move the body. If you find *the* way, you have run into resistance. Form is a delicate balance of confidence and curiosity. Your confidence stems from your trust and your physiological and neurological integration of the postures, alignments and techniques. Your curiosity stems from the fundamental aliveness that you bring to your practice. Together, these move you to continually learn more and more about yourself and how to engage your training.

Resistance as Breaks in the Posture and Alignment of Your Mind

Proper form as understood and practiced in BMT is articulated through the joining of body and mind into precise movements and expressions of each exercise. The proper posture and alignment of your mind has to do with your attention. Proper form requires that your attention remain focused. Your mental form is articulated through the focus of your attention on the alignment, posture and technique of your physical articulation of the movement. Your attention closely follows each movement. Your mind is focused without distractions when your body-mind is embodying and articulating proper form.

Mental distraction is one of the largest forms of resistance. Your conditioned mind will resist the "inner posture and alignment" of focusing your attention upon your body-mind. Your habituation will actively resist being engaged with the present movements of the body once the neurological and muscular integration occurs. In other words, once you have adequately learned something, there is a tendency to no longer focus, and thus you have the opportunity to mentally "check out." This is "learned disengagement." The mind, while spacious, focused and curious when first learning something, reaches a point where it concludes it has adequately mastered the material. Fast along the way of evolving your practice you find your attention suddenly floating somewhere else.

When your attention divorces itself from the immediacy of your training, no further refining of engagement can occur. Your body-mind has been split. When this separation occurs the practice that is most useful is to notice what pulled your attention away from the immediacy of the movement's posture, alignment and technique. Once you have labeled this you start over. Connect with the core intentions of Body-Mind-Moment Training and then establish a conscious relationship with your breath. Then return to working with your form.

Beginners may need to do this process in between sets, while more experienced practitioners will be able to accomplish this mid-set. The more experienced and the more disciplined your practice, the faster you will be able to realign your mind's posture and thus your engagement.

Working with Resistance: Sensation's Sticking Points

Sensation introduces the idea of letting go. As your form is refined, your attention can relax into the movement. The posture and alignment of the mind's form is characterized by focus. When the sensation stage of engagement comes online, your attention will adopt a more sophisticated stance toward the moment and your training. This shift can be summarized as "focus meets receptivity." Your attention is still highly focused as it remains intimately wedded to each movement, however your focus now softens and becomes much more receptive. It is this receptivity that opens up an attunement with your body-mind. What was once a small object to focus your attention upon opens up into a field of vibrant sensation.

An important point not yet discussed is the three basic perspectives available to us, and the one that BMT privileges. The first perspective of the three is first-person. First-person perspective is articulated with "I," "me" and "mine." The second type is second-person. This is articulated through "you," and is didactic in nature. This perspective is intrinsically conversational. Finally, we have third-person perspective, which is inhabited any time we look at something objectively.

These three basic perspectives are available to us throughout each of the stages of engagement, however BMT privileges the first-person perspective. This is especially important in the sensation stage of engagement because the purpose of this training is to subjectively inhabit your training. The purpose is not necessarily to describe sensations objectively or to converse with various parts of yourself. While these are all welcome within your discipline, the central drive is toward greater first-person inhabitation of your body-mind in the moment[28].

Given that we are granting a privilege to the subjective first-person perspective in our training, creating a second-or third-person relationship with sensations is considered a form of resistance in this stage of engagement. Objectively looking at your sensations and treating them as an "it" creates a separation between you and that which you are. "It is hot," "It is painful," "It is really blissful" and "It is intense" all exhibit examples of this third-person perspective. Similarly, talking to your sensations creates unnecessary separation. "You are so hot," "You are painful," and "You are so blissful," all exhibit this second-person perspective and relationship to the sensations emerging. These second-

and third-person perspectives are distinctly different from the first-person perspective of experiencing the heat as an articulation of who you are in the present moment. "I am heat," "I am bliss," and "I am intensity" are all articulations of this first-person perspective. Again, the sensation stage of engagement is aimed at refining your first-person experience of training. The objectification of your sensations, or any type of dialogue with the sensations as they are arising, is a resistance to embodying the fullness of yourself and your training.

The sensation stage embodies a new type of volition in in which you let go of your conventional ways of controlling both yourself and your training. Resistance-based control transitions to participatory-based control. Influence and control are grounded in and animated by participating with what is already unfolding. This is different from the conventional self's preference to control, based on its own conditioning regardless of what is actually emerging. This is resistance-based control.

This can have a number of causes: failure to rest your full trust in a particular movement philosophy, attachment to your ego's habituated resistance as a means of control, as well as a fear of losing control. Ultimately, once the proper form has been adopted, it is a matter of discipline, practice and simply letting go into the natural process of engagement. While letting go is simple, it is this simplicity that makes it so difficult for your conventional sense of self. In fact, letting go is impossible for the conventional self. Its means of control is dependent upon struggling with what is, not Surrendering and participating with what is. Thus the sensation stage, especially in its more mature expressions, takes an important step beyond the ego's habituated struggle.

Keeping yourself in a prescriptive relationship to form is a common example of resistance while establishing the sensation stage. Instead of embodying the form's immediate sensations, you and the movement remain separate and distinct. You and your body are two entities in which you, the volitional intelligence, are telling the body what to do, and what not to do. The sensation stage embodies a highly integrated body-mind in which this novel emergent is the volitional guiding intelligence. While a prescriptive relationship is necessary for mastering form, this way of relating to your training must be outgrown through disciplined, wholehearted engagement. As practice develops and unfolds, your ability to trust the moment, your training philosophy, and ultimately you, will grow. This development slowly releases the resistance to letting go and allows the prescriptive or controlling relationship to form to be held lightly, eventually leading to a spontaneous release.

"Hardened," or forced, attention is another expression of resistance. While this may have been necessary to master the form stage, this strong mental focus can become a hindrance as it expresses an inability to let go, release and trust the natural unfolding of the process. Forcing your attention accentuates your conventional volitional capacities and reinforces the necessity for added effort. Softening your focus and allowing your attention to broaden can help spark your ability to let go to the spontaneity of your body-mind.

Another form of resistance in this stage is the attachment to enjoyable experiences and the avoidance of painful experiences. With the emergence of the capacity to let go, blissful and enjoyable experiences become much more available to your body-mind. Similarly, letting go opens up your body-mind's ability to inhabit pain.

When you experience either end of this spectrum, your habituated self will most likely become triggered or activated. Attachment to the enjoyable, which often manifests in a subtle or "covert" plan to recreate the pleasurable experiences severs the relationship with the moment and fractures the heart of BMT. Similarly, avoiding the painful dimensions to training is exhibited in a pervasive agenda to avoid experiencing pain. This agenda to avoid results in a contracted expression of training as avoidance. In either case—attachment to pleasure or avoidance of pain —BMT regresses to body-mind "manipulation" training as the connection to the moment is lost.

When your embodied connection with the present moment is lost, you have severed yourself from the source of your Excellence. What is left to guide (or more accurately, misguide) your training is the habituated conditioning of your past. Practitioners are often best suited by reconnecting with BMT's core intention (and its two basic dimensions) and engaging with stage one to reconnect with their breath as it is arising in the moment. Without cultivating and refining your body-mind's capacity to remain rooted in and intimately attuned with the present moment, stage three and all stages beyond it will be largely impossible to enact and explore as a practitioner.

A central point is to not attempt to get rid of these agendas as they are part of the natural functioning of your body-mind. A feature of your evolving engagement is the growth and expansion of your capacity to include more. As such, it is useful to focus on integrating and including the parts of yourself that do resist pain and attach to pleasure. Getting rid of these dimensions of yourself is just another layer of struggle further capturing you into your habituated self. When you allow space for your conditioning to arise freely without compulsively acting from habit, you will experience the greater fullness of who you are. The core intentions of BMT are aimed at connecting you with the parts of yourself that transcend your conditioning around pleasure and pain.

The more you train and practice wholeheartedly the closer you will come to arriving at that which is fundamentally unconditioned, which brings with it the next stage of engagement: Being. Working with the resistance of attachment to pain and pleasure is a process of continual refinement. The more you practice, the more you will see and be able to liberate yourself from ultimately embodying the core intentions of BMT with greater fullness.

Working with Resistance: Being, and the Identification with Doing

All resistance in the Being stage is rooted in the unconscious identification with doing. That is to say your moment-to-moment creation of a self-concept is largely dictated by the activity of your body-mind. While this is not necessarily inaccurate, as your self system's identity certainly depends upon what you do, as your training shifts to this stage the view and process of your conventional self is found to be incomplete. Your conditioned tendency to define yourself through what you do is your primary resistance to stepping consistently into the domain of Being.

Surrendering to Being is qualitatively distinct from the capacity to let go embodied in the sensation stage because that which is Surrendered to is not attached to any activity at all. While both transcend your conventional conditioning and sense of self, Being transcends your relative body-mind entirely. Sensation's letting go hands the authoring agency over to the activity of the spontaneous body-mind. Being's Surrender hands the authoring agency over to itself, which quietly transcends all activity.

When the field of Being is first glimpsed, an attachment to doing is typically animated. This form of resistance is "doing" The Leap. The infinite field of Being is explicitly sought. The fundamental problem here is the continued over-identification with doing. By attempting to "do" The Leap, the practitioner is attempting the impossible (as doing and Being point to two different realms). Thus far your training has been largely if not entirely immersed in the relative domain. With Being, your training is stepping beyond this domain into the transcendent. Fundamentally, there is nothing you can "do" to "be."

The prescription for making The Leap has long been varying forms of meditation (or contemplation, from the Western view) in which the prescription for doing is so simplistic that eventually your conventional body-mind gives up in frustration. It is in this frustrated release that genuine Surrender is experienced and the realm of Being is revealed to the practitioner.

"Doing" meditation is often considered to be a misunderstanding in and of itself. While there are many things that can be done at various stages of meditation practice that can be useful for practitioners, these are simply handrails along the way leading to the release and Surrender we are investigating here. Meditation is in actuality not any kind of "doing" but is itself the seat of Being manifested through practice. Meditation at its heart is *about* Being. All prescriptions to "do" meditation are exercises that when carried through to their end (that is, the exercises are dropped and all habituated activity ceases) results in true meditation.

Eventually your strength training, employing the techniques and technology of BMT, results in the loosening of your identification with doing. When all techniques are Surrendered, The Leap to that which is present all along naturally reveals itself to the heart of the practitioner; Being is known intimately.

Another common form of resistance to evolving one's relationship to Being is getting stuck in not-doing. Often The Leap is initially experienced during periods of inactivity and rest in between sets. As attention naturally opens, and the body releases tension and begins the recovery process from the previous set, you may access brief states of Being. In this state it is easy to get stuck in the simple unbounded joy of sitting on the bench. Your training can become fragmented and will lose its flow if you get stuck in this state between sets. While this has a number of physiological consequences, the underlying problem is that Being becomes known only through the lens of inactivity or non-action. It is important that you follow the flow and rhythm of your training to facilitate the discovery of Being's fundamental ground regardless of the type of action performed.

Another type of resistance is the imposing of preferences *upon* Being. Most commonly this takes form as the enjoyable nature of Being is conflated with the content of your experience. While some of these experiences will be some of the most precious gifts your conventional self has ever known, this does not mean that all your training from this fourth stage is going to be universally blissful.

Being is limitless because of its fundamental liberation from all preferences. This transcendence of preferences enables the fullness of all experiences that come and go without limitation. By attaching preferences and attempting to recreate or manufacture enjoyable training experiences, you sever the connection with the transcendent seat of Being. Similarly, to avoid pain and suffering in your training severs your connection.

The further you penetrate into the heart of your training the more obvious Being becomes. While your first encounters feel as though something new is being added to your training, as training matures Being is known as something that is not added, it just is. You have been resting in this timeless seat all along; the only "addition" is your realization of the fundamental seat of your unconditioned self. When you animate your training from Being you are enveloping and integrating your body-mind and the moment.

Access to the reservoir of Being's transcendence can facilitate extraordinary feats of strength, power, endurance and grace in your training. These training feats are largely governed by the synthesis of your spontaneous body-mind with the transcendent nature of Being. These extraordinary feats are activities that your conditioned self is drawn to possessing. This form of resistance to Being is again rooted in an attachment to doing, although in this particularly charged case, we are pointing to doing actions that are extraordinary, that is to say, they transcend the normal means by which the conditioned self moves and accomplishes things in the world.

The fundamental rub here is your conventional self's attachment to these actions. When you get attached to these feats, your habituated self will want to own and possess them so that it can control and leverage them. They cannot be possessed and governed by a lesser integrative structure. Your conditioned self cannot in any way, shape or form possess that which stems from the unconditioned.

There are two important points here. To attempt to control these capacities often results in a regression into earlier stages of engagement as the connection with the moment becomes weakened. If this attempt is sought by the practitioner they are no longer practicing BMT, as this commitment fractures the core orientation of BMT and largely unplugs the practitioner from the present moment. While there are no good places to get stuck, this one is particularly nasty in its ability to capture years of people's training and lives.

Second, a more sophisticated conditioned self can leverage strategies for manufacturing states in which genuine Surrender can emerge thus gaining access to the capacity to perform extraordinary feats. When this "state manufacturing" is adequately learned, the practitioner begins to leverage transcendent states and functioning to serve his conditioned self. This is also an extremely difficult sticking point to grow from because the conditioning often results in exacerbating suffering both in the practitioner's personal life and training.

Finally, the last form of resistance is getting stuck in a third-person relationship to Being. Instead of embodying Being from the first-person perspective, it is common for practitioners to get stuck in looking at "it" objectively. Just as in the relationship to sensation, BMT privileges the first-person perspective.

Working with Resistance: Mystery and the Trap of Knowing

The principle resistance to the Mystery stage of engagement is knowing. Working with resistance at this stage of training means to investigate and untangle yourself from deep-seated assumptions around knowing. The experience of knowing is the antithesis of engaging your training as the Mystery. Thus, just about all forms of knowing obscure this level of engagement. The central resistance is the assumption that you know who you are.

To shift beyond glimpses of the Mystery stage of engagement you must go to the root assumption here: that you know who you are. While you can continue to know yourself in more conventional ways, fundamentally you are not attached to any of the answers as you penetrate the heart of who you are. This knowing, which is actually a realization of not-knowing, is the only type of knowledge to rest within during this stage. Again, conventional knowledge about who you are, what you are doing, how you are training, etc., remains perfectly intact and functional, but you no longer fall into the trap of believing that this is fundamentally who you are.

Training from the seat of Being is the central objective of the preceding stage of engagement, however it is now the obstacle and resistance to be overcome if the Mystery is to be fully enacted in your training. Training from limitless non-doing holds an assumption where oneself is known as the ever-present witness or infinite ground of Being. As such, this confidence in one's selfhood and identity is a major obstacle to work with for refining your training.

You may experience the Mystery as a subtle fleeting uncertainty that you hardly notice, you may experience a pervasive silence amidst your training, or you may suddenly find yourself doubting. Your development in this stage will closely depend upon your ability to Surrender into not-knowing (or non-knowing). Your conditioned self experiences anxiety as this silent empty void, unknowable through and through, reveals itself.

Two common sticking points for this stage are getting stuck in questions, and getting stuck in answers. Getting stuck in questions suggests that you can know the Mystery. The illusion and conditioning that you can know remains intact and thus you continue to present questions and attempt to answer them. Body-Mind-Moment practitioners are encouraged to assess where their questions originate.

Some questions are an articulation of your conditioned self attempting to gain control after an encounter with Mystery. These questions are often intellectual in nature and shift easily from one question to the next. If your questions are encouraging you to reflect back on an experience you already had, you are caught in questioning. In your training you will suddenly find your body doing one thing, your mind pondering something else and your training largely divorced from the present moment. Practitioners without as much experience may fall into this habituated pattern and in its unconscious familiarity remain stuck in various forms of inquiry that divorce their body-mind from the present moment.

If, however, your question is persistent and its energy is drawing your body-mind to investigate the direct experience in this moment, then you are caught in a question that is leading you into the Mystery. Both forms of inquiry are expressions of resistance to the Mystery in your training, however one is headed directly away from realizing your affinity with this unknowable ground and the other is headed toward your direct inhabitation of the Mystery.

Getting caught in answers has two different expressions that are generally dependent upon where the question originates. If the question is a surface-level inquiry, your conditioned mind will become entrapped in surface-level answers about what might have been, what could be, what was, and so on. If the question stems from a genuine seat of doubt, your answer will reverberate in your body-mind. This is not a discursive question that comes and goes; this type of question stems from a pervasive uncertainty that is you.

Regardless of how rooted and embodied an answer is, it still remains a separation and resistance to the Mystery. You reside "over here" with the question and answer about the Mystery that resides "over there." This relationship fails at Surrendering into the Mystery that you are. As you mature into this stage of your training, you come to realize the void and unknowable emptiness at your source.

You train with a great doubt at the center of who you are, and you relate to your training as a great unknown. The Mystery spreads from the heart of your own witness to the fullness of your activity and all that is arising around your body-mind in the moment. It is from this Mystery that true confidence in your training stems, and the genuine seat of confidence for your highest expressions of performance resides. If your highest expressions of your performance and Excellence are not born from the radical immediacy of Mystery then you have yet to inhabit and articulate the most central call for Excellence in your life.

Working with Resistance: Attaching to the Dual in Non-Duality

Resistance, as it pertains to the non-dual suchness of your training, organizes around dualities. Duality itself is the resistance to be worked with. The dualism to be released is between self and other.

This is not a matter of looking at someone and thinking, "They are essentially no different than me," or, "The witness that looks through my eyes is the same that perceives through their eyes." While these may be important conceptual musings, they miss the direct territory. The non-dual is not the content of unitive thoughts. The realization of the non-dual ground that you already are requires you to let go of the habituated contraction around you completely. When you do so, you find that your direct immediate experience prior to any thought has no duality. As thought arrises, there is no duality. As thought falls away, there is no duality.

The "other" that you look at from "your" body-mind's eyes is experienced directly as your own first-person subjective seat of awareness. While the "other" remains "out there" in relationship to your conditioned self, you experience the "other" as yourself directly, without any mediation. Self and other remain useful relative distinctions, and you can still easily navigate these apparent dualities, however the truth of your direct experience is that you know yourself firsthand as the other. Self and other become "not two."

The distinctions here may be helpful, but only to a point, because we are creating a duality between what is dual and what is non-dual. This is necessary for our discussion, but from the perspective of the non-dual even this distinction does not hold up. Duality itself is the non-duality we are attempting to point at. Here we arrive at a paradox. What remains for us is our practice, our disciplined engagement with our training. The more wholeheartedly you engage with yourself and your training the more prone you are to stumbling into the realization of the non-dual. The further you carry your training, the more expansive your expression of this non-dual condition. It is to this aim that we are all called, to turn toward our training and engage moment to moment, without hesitation. Engage, engage, engage! This is true sound of the resistance we press into as we train.

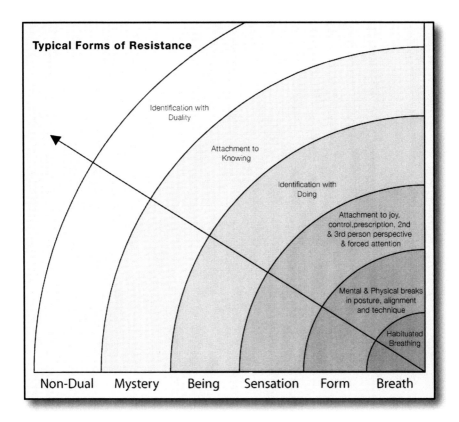

Chapter Fourteen

The Process of Execution

In the last two chapters we took a look at the interior dimension of engagement and resistance as it pertains to Body-Mind-Moment Training. You now have a road map of where to place your attention, how your sense of selfhood shifts and evolves and how your volitional faculty develops and refines as your engagement with practice progresses. Next we will turn our attention to some of the external dimensions of this practice. While the interior dimension of engagement focuses on *how* to engage, the exterior dimension of BMT will begin to focus on *what* to do. Here you will learn the basic principles of movement, the Macro and MicroCycles that leverage and integrate the core modalities of movement, and the U-Theory of Performance, as we begin to explore the implications of BMT on performance.

Principles of Movement

Your body has two primary dimensions in movement. Therefore, BMT also has two basic principles of movement: contraction and extension. Movement tends to emphasize either a contracting (or tensing) dimension, or it emphasizes an extending (or releasing) dimension. Strength training in its conventional forms typically only emphasizes the contraction dimension of movement. If a practice is to be integrative in its essential nature it must embody and address *both* dimensions of movement. BMT accomplishes this through two different means: the MacroCycle and the MicroCycle. To place these into context, let us first take a look at the U-Theory of Performance.

U-Theory of Performance

Many people assume performance to be a linear progression. The basic premise is that as skill and experience grow so does performance. This linear relationship between performance, skill and experience is largely related only to the early phases of the development of performance. Beyond this preliminary[29] linear progression lies the U-Theory of Performance, a three-phase orientation to the overall development of new performance capacities.

The first stage culminates in an exclusive orientation of one of the primary dimensions of movement. In strength training this beginning phase is the contraction dimension. In yoga[30] this stage exhibits an exclusive focus on extension. With either dimension of movement, the initial stage is defined by an exclusive focus on the leading dimension. The sole purpose of the movement is to express the greatest contraction (as in strength training) or the greatest extension (as in yoga) within a prescribed set of movements.

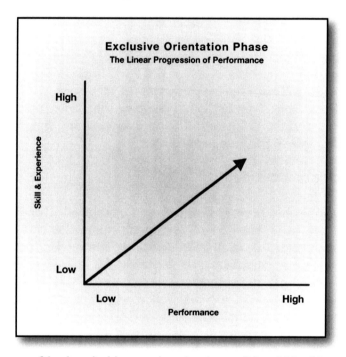

The degree of body-mind integration that is possible within this exclusive orientation stage is quite limited, however the body-mind naturally seeks to integrate the two fundamental dimensions of movement within each moment. This is the inherent gradient to which your body-mind is bound. The ego's predisposition however is to attach to performance standards in this beginning stage, limiting your ability to Surrender to the inherent gradient your body-mind seeks to align with, which ultimately increases performance capacities.

The second stage of the U-Theory of Performance is the intersection stage. This intermediate step brings the two fundamental dimensions of movement into contact with one another *within* the moment. The two basic dimensions of movement are polarities. As a result, the unintegrated nervous system's attempt to unite them often inhibits performance standards, at least initially. When a practitioner who has yet to sufficiently integrate their nervous system focuses upon the extension dimension of an exercise, their ability to produce the most powerful contraction is limited. Similarly any focus upon the contraction dimension within a yoga asana (the seat or body position taken during the practice of yoga) initially increases tension and reduces the overall range of motion of the asana.

Practitioners are encouraged to work through these limitations as they move through the intersection stage. A dip in performance is necessary in order to adopt and integrate a new modality of movement, one that integrates both fundamental modalities within the movement regardless of the emphasis. While performance is compromised in this stage, the foundation and platform for a new level of synergy is being established.

The third stage of the U-Theory of Performance is integration. Here we find a novel synergy of the two fundamental movement modalities that supersedes the previous peaks in performance. For example, an asana in yoga will move toward the perfection of the movement as the body-mind learns to engage and contract the asana's antagonist muscles. For example, in a forward bend the action of contracting and drawing the quadriceps upward on the front of the leg triggers the hamstrings to release and extend more fully through a process called reciprocal inhibition. This increases the forward bend. As the practitioner learns to isolate and engage antagonist contractions the asana spontaneously refines in ways not possible when focusing only upon the extension dimension. Therefore, the forward bend will not open as fully when the practitioner focuses solely upon stretching and extending her hamstrings.

Similarly, in strength training a new territory of performance opens up in the integration stage. Peak performance in strength training can be defined by three characteristics. The first is moving resistance through a controlled range of motion with the most amount of speed. This first factor can be summarized as the body-mind's *fastest range of motion* when given a resistance. The second factor is a *strong container*, which means there are no breaks in form, and the fastest range of motion follows a clear groove in which the movement does not deviate. High levels of performance outside of this structure are not expressions of peak performance but instead are often expressions of physical and/or mental limitations, which create predispositions to injuries. These presumed high levels of performance outside of a strong container should be carefully examined, especially as you explore the higher reaches of performance. Finally, your peak performance flowers with the third element: *the least amount of effort.* While the principle discipline requires immense levels of effort, your highest expressions of these emergent capacities reside in the repetition(s) in which you perform the movement with the least amount of effort. United, your fastest range of motion, with the least amount of effort, within a strong container brings forth your expression of peak performance.

Peak Performance Triad

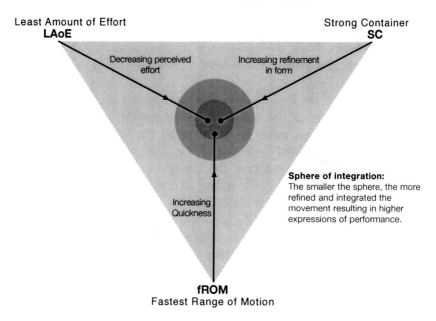

Least Amount of Effort
LAoE

Strong Container
SC

Decreasing perceived
effort

Increasing refinement
in form

Sphere of integration:
The smaller the sphere, the more refined and integrated the movement resulting in higher expressions of performance.

Increasing
Quickness

fROM
Fastest Range of Motion

For example, this is what it looks like when you have a ballistic, explosive strength training exercise pushing out against a pneumatic resistance in the integration phase. First we have a strong container. The bones of the hand and wrist remain in alignment with the elbow so all the force generated through the chest and triceps muscles is channelled with great efficiency into the resistance. Similarly the hips conduct power and stability from the legs and feet, which hold the genesis of the movement. The power originates in the foot and is transferred up the ankle and through the legs, ultimately aligned with the chest and triceps muscles. The fastest range of motion is displayed first through starting power. This starting power, or the maximal force generated when beginning a movement, emphasizes the contraction dimension of movement. This increases the body-mind's capacity for speed and quickness. Generating the most pronounced starting power is not created through the most effort. By creating the least amount of effort the movement simultaneously inhabits both release and openness that optimizes conductivity and minimizes resistance in the antagonist muscles, thus increasing the amount of force generated. This sets the body-mind to exhibit the fastest range of motion: progressive acceleration. Progressively moving faster and faster through a range of movement culminating in a peak output just as the arm has reached full extension. It is through the complete release and extension of the arm that the highest degrees of power and force are brought to fruition. Throughout this movement maximal force is generated with the least amount of effort.

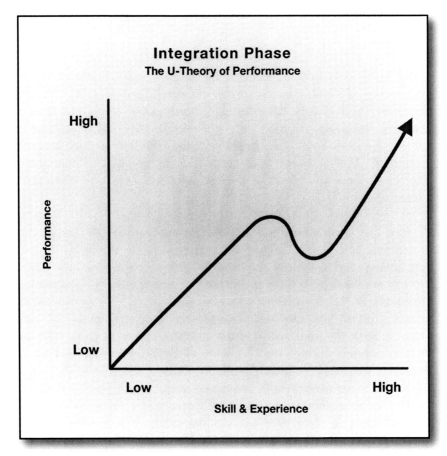

The integration stage provides the unique synthesis of the two basic dimensions of movement necessary to access the fastest range of motion with the least amount of effort within a strong container for movement. Surrendering to your training in this fashion relaxes your body-mind, resulting in greater fluidity and conductivity of will and effort, as well as a profound physiological release. This integration brings contraction and release into a synergistic balance that embodies performance levels unattainable by the exclusive focus upon contraction itself.

MacroCycles - The Basic Integration of Movement Modalities

Strength training is fundamentally a fragmented discipline if it remains solely focused on contracting the muscles during each exercise. While there is a natural release and extension following each set, an intentional cooperation with this process is needed if your body-mind is to continue to engage intimately with the moment. Strength training as an Integral Practice must actively participate with both fundamental principles of movement.

The MacroCycles in BMT provide the fundamental framework for the integration of both movement modalities. The MacroCycles are performed immediately following (or shortly after) the completion of your last repetition. As soon as you complete your last repetition, or release the resistance, you begin to shift the orientation of your movement. During a set your orientation is toward the contraction dimension. Once you complete the last repetition your orientation shifts to extension.

If you are contracting the muscle groups responsible for *pushing* movements (chest and triceps) your extension phase would focus upon lengthening and releasing the muscle groups responsible for *pulling* movements (back and biceps). Whatever muscle group(s) you worked principally in the contraction phase of your practice determines what muscle group(s) you emphasize during the extension phase of your practice. Both the contraction phase and the extension phase of your training progress through the U-Theory of Performance outlined above. Beginners will focus exclusively upon contraction, followed by extension. Advanced practitioners will integrate both within each phase of movement. Practitioners can be at different stages along the U given predispositions in their practice and discipline. It is possible that an advanced strength trainer adopting BMT expresses and articulates the integration stage during the contraction phase, but given a lack of practice he may be at the exclusive orientation stage during the extension phase. While these different levels of competence are possible, practitioners are encouraged to seek a balance.

The MacroCycle

While the term "set" has been used thus far as a group of repetitions of an exercise, moving forward it will refer to the completion of both the contraction *and* the extension phase in BMT.

The basic formula for the MacroCycle is to balance the time expended within each phase of movement. If you spend approximately 45 seconds in the contraction phase you would spend about 45 seconds in the extension phase. This is a preliminary formula that is recommended for beginners only and should not necessarily be followed by intermediate or advanced practitioners. Use it to get you started, but as your engagement evolves you will want to shift away from prescribed formulas and move toward an intuitive feel. Consequently your MacroCycle may end up being balanced during the first set only to move to a 1 to 3 ratio during the second set, with the third set expressing a 2 to 1 ratio.

MacroCycle Examples:		
	Contraction Phase	Extension Phase
Set 1:	45 seconds	45 seconds
Set 2:	30 seconds	90 seconds
Set 3:	40 seconds	20 seconds

If you notice that one dimension is lagging behind the other you are encouraged to spend more time working with the neglected dimension.

Engagement and the MacroCycles

Each phase moves through its own engagement continuum outlined in chapters ten and eleven. While each phase is most commonly navigated from the same stage of engagement, it is possible to have one phase originate from a different stage of engagement. For example, a yoga practitioner may be working principally on the Form stage of engagement in her contraction phase yet be firmly rooted in the Being stage of engagement during her extension phase.

Engagement Example:

Contraction Phase	Extension Phase
Breath	Breath
Form	Form
Sensation	Sensation
Being	**Being**
Mystery	Mystery
Non Dual	Non Dual

Beginners will often have some variance between the level of engagement they bring to each phase, given their body-mind's predisposition toward one of the fundamental movement dimensions. As your training unfolds, the lagging dimension often quickly catches up to your leading phase. It is important to note that the process often privileges one dimension. That is to say you may have a peak experience, a sudden spontaneous shift in one phase of your practice, while the complimentary phase remains largely unchanged. These shifts in your training are best handled by Surrendering to the process or trusting the spontaneous rhythms your training may take. This is a natural part of the process of your training: adapting and integrating new stages of engagement.

Exceptions to Surrendering

There are three central aspects that may indicate that your body-mind is ready to follow when a peak experience (regardless of whether it is pleasurable in nature, painful or a mix) emerges in your training. The first is a positive exploratory attitude toward the peak experience. If fear outweighs your curiosity it may be best to investigate this throughly in a reflective process outside of your training. The second marker is whether you feel the peak experience is increasing your risk for injury. If your peak experience has brought forth a loss of control where your movements lie outside your strong container it is not appropriate to Surrender to the natural movement of this experience. The third marker, which is much more difficult to work, is when the process is interfering with the functioning of your life outside of your training.

It is safe to assume that every practitioner, with the right discipline and perseverance, will encounter large peak experiences in their training at least once in their life. These periods can be extremely challenging and can last up to several months in some cases. The four areas used to assess yourself are friends, family, intimate relationships and job performance. If these areas of your life are deteriorating, the process unfolding may be too challenging. In cases where your functioning has been significantly impaired it is useful to investigate whether this process correlates with any stressful precipitating factors in your life. Your training is a microcosm of your life.

Exceptions to Surrendering

1. Fear outweighs curiosity to go into the peak experience.

2. A loss of control places you in greater risk for injury.

3. The peak experience is significantly interfering with functioning in life outside of training (friendships, family, intimate relationships and job performance).

MicroCycles

MicroCycles are a foundation for intermediate practitioners. MicroCycles facilitate practitioners as they refine their nervous system to begin to articulate the third integration stage. While practitioners in the integration stage synergistically enact the two fundamental movement modalities within the moment, MicroCycles are shortened periods of emphasis upon one dimension, followed by emphasis on the other. There are many different ways to leverage MicroCycles, but one common method for moving your practice from the intersection stage to the integration stage is to employ both movement modalities in each phase of the lift. Thus, during pushing movements the practitioner emphasizes the contraction dimension of movement. As the contraction phase progresses past its midpoint the extension dimension of movement is emphasized. Similarly, as the weight is lowered during the eccentric movement, the concentric dimension is emphasized, followed by the extension dimension as the repetition nears the transition between lowering and lifting the resistance.

These MicroCycles begin to refine the nervous system to hold these two movement modalities closer together. As such we find that the body-mind grows in its capacity for performance and engagement. Transitions between concentric and eccentric movements can occur with much greater speed, precision and intentional engagement through the use of MicroCycles. Within each repetition the fierce will and effort deployed at the bottom of the lift will seamlessly transmute into a Surrender and release. This intrinsically aligns the body-mind with the moment.

MicroCycles and Performance

Let us take a look at elite performance ballistic training (where the principle objective is to produce the fastest, most powerful complete movement with the most energy-efficient form). This is the core skill set of most elite athletes, so if you want to become one you will need to master MicroCycles and eventually the integration stage in your athletic discipline. BMT is an advanced tool to cultivate the necessary neurological and muscular systems and psychological foundation for the highest levels of performance.

One example of a MicroCycle in ballistic training is what I call the "Ballistic MicroCycle," where the first part of the movement emphasizes the contraction phase while integrating the extension phase as described above. This optimizes the critical performance metric known as starting power. This can be seen in a medicine ball throw when the ball is held in front of the chest and the body-mind is recruited to press and throw the ball into a wall as forcefully as possible. Movement starts and reaches maximal exertion as quickly as possible, requiring strong contractions in the prime movers (legs and arms); stabilizing muscle groups also contract, improving the conductivity of energy up the legs through the torso and out the arms. All the while opposing muscle groups relax, thus minimizing resistance to the force generated. This maximal starting power happens within the first two inches of movement as the medicine ball is forcefully pressed away from the chest.

As the movement shifts into its second phase, this forceful contraction and integrated extension creates a phenomena called progressive acceleration. This essential feature of performance progressively moves the medicine ball faster and faster away from the body the further away the ball gets from the chest. This culminates in the ball being released from the hands with the arms fully extended where the muscles of the arms momentarily release. This maximizes power output. Here, at the peak of extension and release, where all energy has been focused and expended, the third phase of movement begins where the arms return to their starting position, drawing back the medicine ball back into the chest. For ballistic training this means drawing back as swiftly as possible, emphasizing the contraction dimension. As the returning movement approaches its end, the contraction phase engages to decelerate and control the movement to begin deploying the beginning contraction of the next movement. This minimizes the transition time between repetitions.

The Intersection of Engagement and Performance

The U-Theory of Performance looks at how you move and perform largely from an exterior perspective, which means we can look at the way you are moving and determine which modality you are engaging. The U-Theory looks at how your nervous system relates to the two fundamental modalities of movement and the complexity within which you move through the three basic stages: exclusive orientation, intersection and integration. However, this external perspective is incomplete and fragmented without integrating the interior perspective on your training: the Stages of Engagement. Your subjective experience is the interior dimension. These are subjective truths that largely only your direct first-person experience can disclose. If someone wants to know this part of you with a high degree of accuracy they are wise to engage in discourse with you. It is through this discourse, this exchange of interiors, that someone can come to know your subjective experience. Together, the U-Theory of Performance and the Stages of Engagement provide a useful means of evaluating your training and fueling integrated development, as well as performance gains.

Just as in the conscious engagement with your discipline, the foundation of all performance is your breath and form. When your body-mind ceases integrating your breathing and movement, performance and engagement plummet. Similarly, the moment your form breaks, performance falls and the qualitative engagement within your body-mind necessarily follows. These are the foundations of performance and engagement. They are prerequisites for the fullest and most refined expression of your Excellence.

Breath and form are essential for optimal gains in the exclusive orientation phase of the U-Theory of Performance. To explore beyond this performance envelope, to reach further into your greater developmental unfolding, you must establish a clear, consistent engagement with sensation. It is the sensation stage of engagement that enables practitioners to work with great skill with contraction and extension. The sensation stage enables practitioners to move through the intersection phase into the integration phase where we find a new level of performance previously unattainable, but it is only the minimum prerequisite to shift beyond the exclusive orientation's performance limitations. Engagement beyond the sensation stage facilitates more refined and pronounced performance gains as the integration phase matures, bringing forth a greater embodiment and enactment of training, competition and life.

Chapter Fifteen

The Paradox of
Peak Performance

The Fragmented Approach

What is peak performance? Is it setting a new record, winning at the highest levels, performing at your best, exceeding someone else's best?

While these are conventional standards of peak performance they point to interpretations that are often fragmented both in their aim and pursuit. The first problem with this approach is the split between the third person perspective of your body as an object and the subjective realm of your direct first person experience (when it is ignored in the pursuit of making your body perform). This seemingly innocent divorce between your subjective and objective dimensions of the self splinters your body-mind's capacity to perform at your best. Invariably when this split occurs you are left with two parts, not an integrated whole. Your Excellence does not stem from fragmentation but instead greater and greater integration.

When this fragmentation occurs, consciously or unconsciously, you will make a choice as to which part you value more. If you happen to subscribe to the predominant paradigm on performance, you mistakenly value the measurable objective dimension of yourself *over* the sphere of your direct subjective experience. When the body-mind is split into a mind looking at a body, there is a tendency to treat part of yourself as an object and to devalue and dismiss the realm of your subjective experience. As such you may be familiar with "pushing *it* harder," "commanding *your body* to do more," telling your body to "stop being so weak" pleading with *it* to "hold up" to the demands you have forced, invited or created in your training. All the while the subjective interior experience is largely ignored.

The second problem of the unconscious pursuit of externally measured performance is the split between the pre-personal and personal stages of functioning. Human development can be divided into three stages. The pre-personal stage in which the sense of self is yet to be adequately formed. The second is the personal stage where the individuated and autonomous self is established and maintained. Finally, the third stage, the trans-personal, extends beyond the conventional self. A wider sense of identity and a new set of functional capacities emerges that transcends yet includes the personal and pre-personal stages.

Too often the externally measured paradigm's approach to performance results in prolonged and contracted pre-personal stages of functioning. When pre-personal injunctions are leveraged to enhance objectively measured performance metrics the emerging sphere of personhood is denied in key ways. This fragmentation coupled with the subscription to exclusively objective measurements of all types yields tremendous self sacrifice. This tends to stunt overall growth and performance. Alternatively (although rare), self-sacrifice can also blossom into a legitimate path to an authentic resolution of this fragmentation, which inherently supports increasing performance capacities. That is the central difficulty many people remain trapped in: self-sacrifice both holds you back *and* is the gateway through which all of your greater potential resides.

With a fragmented aim and approach to performance, practitioners largely tend to stunt the greater unfolding of their performance capacities. It is through a more integrative perspective and approach that you can skillfully leverage your core impulse to sacrifice yourself for performance to authentically support your emergent Excellence.

The Double-Edged Sword of Self-Sacrifice

The good news is that when self-sacrifice embodies Surrender, and is given to something greater than your own personal performance and preference, ironically it *then* unfolds within a new sphere of possibility. The negative side of self-sacrifice is when it embodies submission. It is this core distinction that sends the practitioner in two different directions.

Submission can, and often does, initially produce performance gains. This traps many practitioners as they become attached to the performance results gained through submission.

Submission has two distinct features that are often problematic. The first is that it is largely pre-personal, and embraces perspectives, intentions and actions that do not adequately acknowledge the personhood (or emerging personhood) of the practitioner. The second problem is the divorce from your interior subjective felt experience. Here the practitioner's own interior wisdom of how best to perform and train is ignored. In these cases we discover that the "I" has been largely severed from an agency worthy of consideration. As a result, the sense of self that is most identified with is the objective, measurable part of oneself. The "I" becomes an "it."

When you start to treat yourself as an "it," you depersonalize yourself. Your interior begins to get marginalized and devalued. How you authentically feel, what your most true motivations are, how alive you feel in your life and training only matter so much as whether your felt subjective experience holds any perceived influence upon how well you objectively perform. When your subjective experience is marginalized to that which is objectively measurable there is little room for your authentic "I."

The sad reality is that some of the top athletes in the world hate their sport. Even more painful is the millions of practitioners who remain stuck in a similar relationship to their discipline. As a result we find people who hate the process of articulating their peak performance. Unfortunately, the drive for greatness fueled by submission is driving the athlete or practitioner further *away* from his or her own Excellence, even if they may be temporarily *improving*. If this is the greatness sought, we need to seriously reconsider the process through which our aspirations are pursued.

The more skilled and evolved practitioner will learn to embody greater degrees of Surrender, which transcends and includes the sphere of personhood and continually expands the performance horizon in novel ways. The less developed practitioner will learn to embody greater degrees of submission in which more of the sphere of personhood is denied in service of chasing objective performance goals.

While some conventional approaches to performance yield an unbalanced focus upon measurable outcomes, another alternative is common. Conventional perspectives around performance also yield a general avoidance of performance disciplines as a whole. Performance, evaluation and judgement are sensitive topics in human experience. They can quickly give rise to shame, guilt, feelings of inadequacy and lack of self-worth. This is especially the case when so few differentiate between personhood and behavior (performance). These individuals often value their first-person subjective experience over measurable third-person measurements. Just as the first group, who, in an unbalanced fashion overvalued objective measurements and devalued subjective experience, this group is turned off by competition and objective measurement altogether and devalues its importance while elevating its own first-person experience as the true criteria of what really matters. Ultimately the critic is correctly perceiving personhood as being intrinsically worth more than any behavior that can be exhibited. Unfortunately both are often caught in their partiality and do not see the ability to engage both domains, the interior subjective and the exterior measurable, in an integrated fashion that serves a higher aim.

Submission and the Problem of Possession

Submission provides a preliminary approach to improving objective performance metrics but is principally a dissociative process that disposes of or denies large parts of the self. The subjective dimensions of the self are largely not welcomed to participate and engage with the discipline. There is little to no room for the subjective life, as one of the core fears is that this part is weak, unfocused and will harm performance levels. Given this intrinsic conflict, the practitioner loses interior alignment, diverting energy away from the discipline and its highest enactment, which is one liberated from habituated struggle.

The identity of someone who is mostly consumed and governed by submission has one of two expressions. The first involves the self possessing the capacity to submit to a perceived "great other." In this case submission is to something, and in most cases, someone. Self-sacrifice becomes a badge of honor and a central vehicle for the developing ego. This dynamic is particularly challenging and poses many long-term risks.

The second expression in the self system that is governed by submission is identical, with one exception: That which is submitted to is internalized within the self system. In our first constellation, the "great other" is something or someone *outside* of themselves. They place their trust entirely upon this authority and follow their instruction to a "T." The alternative emerges when the self system grows in organizational complexity and imposes imperatives upon themselves without the need of an outside source of authority. That which these practitioners submit to is not someone but most often a knowledge base and approach that belongs to someone else. While these are similar they are distinct, as these positions inhabit different developmental achievements.

Submission to a philosophy or strategy is not the same as to a person. There is a level of refinement and clarity when someone differentiates whether to submit to a person or to their instruction. The latter enables them to begin to consider the instruction in new ways that submission to a person simply misses altogether. For example, submission to a person implies that this individual's perspective is more important than your own and thus submission is to this person's governing influence in its entirety. In contrast, submission to instruction differentiates between the person and what their instruction is. The instruction is held as the governing influence, not the broad range of preferences, moods, expectations and so on that can accompany the person, and are often layered on top of the instruction being provided.

This latter expression of submission is one step away from the personal realm of performance (as opposed to the pre-personal). As the sense of self develops and ultimately transcends and includes a new agency with *more* control, a greater capacity to perform takes center stage. It is important to note that rarely do we find practitioners who are largely governed by submission in a black or white fashion. However, practitioners articulating submission will tend to organize themselves around one of these two core expressions.

For practitioners who feel their center of gravity originates in submission (and for professionals working with performers on various levels) please take note: There is nothing inherently wrong with submission. We have focused on the limitations of submission only to point out the territory that lies beyond this approach. There are situations where submission is the most viable option given the particular dynamics of an individual at that point in time. Fundamentally though, submission lacks the integrity the highest levels of performance require. If you are invested in performance *and* you are largely negotiating yourself and training through submission you will need to challenge yourself to grow beyond this strategy. You are more than obedience and mimicry.

Personhood & Performance

At some point in the course of training and development, the self can grow to a point where selfhood becomes an absolute necessary ally for achievement and performance. These practitioners feel the truth that their interior experience and the subjective seat of their personhood are as important as performance metrics. When *both* are valued the individual can enter into the personal realm of performance.

The personal domain opens up a new performance horizon in several important ways that are not possible to achieve through the approaches intrinsic to submission. Through personal consideration, self-authoring and pleasure we will explore the greater synergy between the body and mind and how these relate to performance. As we will see, this collaborative alliance harnesses greater energy, stronger focus and more attuned alignment. It is through this greater integration of interior and exterior that practitioners are capable of growing into their higher performance capacities.

Personal Consideration

The heart of personal consideration is *personal understanding*. Here the self system embraces preferences and the construction of various strategies and processes through which execution is refined and tailored to the unique gifts and needs your personhood has. You are more in sync with your self system. This attunement with yourself holds and embraces a greater depth of presence, a greater fullness of performance. This is in contrast to the interior divorce and denial embedded within submission.

Your personal understanding enables you to begin to see your *personal conditioning*. While your personal understanding envelops the present moment's desires and preferences, your personal conditioning enables you to come to know your enduring predispositions. Some of these predispositions are chosen while others are largely a function of your historical conditioning. It is through knowing your historical conditioning that you can understand your greatest strengths and weaknesses. As you embrace more of your conditioning you claim new capacities to tailor your training to skillfully work with these dimensions of yourself. The key here is your training can be tailored to you, by you. Expanding your understanding of how you function facilitates performance in ways submission entirely ignores through its devaluation of subjective experience.

Perhaps the most beautiful dimension of personal consideration is *personal insight*. Personal insights are glimpses into the unfolding novelty of you.

There is no one in the world who can see the true depth and possibility of what is to unfold as you. Personal insights are the moments when you suddenly see more, feel more and know more. The fabric of your Being has broken through your conditioning and now temporarily sees a new intersection of you and your discipline. In a way, personal insight enables you to see into your future possibilities. These personal insights must be captured and solidified in your practice. Once the glimpse into your emerging Excellence comes to a close, all that remains is the preceding stage's implicit limitations and ingrained strategies. Integrating personal insights is essential for the continued growth of your performance capacities. Submission largely misses all of this in its subservience to another's instruction. Without the space to allow what is inside to emerge, practitioners will remain enslaved to imitation and obedience. Both are largely pre-personal phenomena.

Self-Authoring

The self system that is self-authoring rests in a strong seat of maturity. As such the apprenticeship is over. The sphere of inclusion is broad as is the careful consideration of your own purpose in the world and why you train, practice and perform the way you do. Self-authorship holds a vision, a personal mission that is completely and entirely unique to you. You hold a confidence, a seat of certainty that can only be discovered, lived, created and actualized through your own body-mind. This felt sense is an ever-growing certainty in which your self-confidence expands, strengthens and refines itself through testing and re-testing the body-mind in the laboratory of practice.

Self-Authoring also brings with it the ability to *self-initiate, correct and evaluate your training.* This does not mean that you do not take in feedback from those around you, but that fundamentally you make the decisions about your program and evaluate your progress. Unlike submission, where the authority resides in someone else or their philosophy and instruction, with self-authoring the guiding agency resides within you and your direct experience, wisdom and insight. You provide yourself with goals and visions, as well as the self-generated values that support and challenge you to enact your greater levels of Excellence. Goals that are defined, managed and measured by the practitioner possess a much more stable coherent synergy between one's subjective interior and one's measured objective exterior.

A third essential aspect of self-authorship is an expanded desire to take responsibility. It is welcomed and even actively sought by practitioners who have access to self-authorship. By expanding this capacity you widen the sphere of engagement and execution. Your "executive self" has emerged and with this part of you is the ability to respond to the demands of training and performance with greater consideration. The envelope of performance capacities therefore expands into new territories.

Pleasure

Practitioners within the personal stage of performance eventually stumble across this single realization: Their objective measurable performance reaches new heights when they feel the most joyous or connected with their discipline. Practitioners perform not out of obligation, but rather out of a desire to enjoy the activity for its own sake. It is here that the practitioner falls in love with practice, both in training and in performance.

Pleasure is at the root of your evolution. To develop is to expand. When your training is wed to pleasure, your performance and your evolution have become integrated and intertwined. Each moment is an experiment into how you can enact your heart's fullest, most liberated pleasure. It is in the intersection of ecstatic movement and radical presence that you stand on the precipice of the trans-personal. The more you merge your body-mind with the moment, the more authentic and refined the articulation of your Excellence. At the same time the more you genuinely give yourself into the present moment in service of performance, the more you realize that the Excellence you are does not belong to you at all.

When adding personhood into the equation a new self-governed agency has emerged. Greater attunement with oneself results in greater alignment and expanded training and performance capacities. As a result the two central limitations of practices and perspectives embedded within the sphere of submission and the pre-personal domain are resolved. The subjective first-person experience can be skillfully integrated with the pursuit of objective measurements of performance, and the inherent splitting from the personal domain and its intrinsic authorship is metabolized and reborn into this new structure of self with greater response-ability.

The Bad News of Personhood

The personal domain is comprised of a series of hard-won evolutionary advances that shift the sphere of performance beyond the limitations of submission, imitation and obedience, but there are liabilities as well. The first is when the features of the personal domain, fears of failure, judgement and acceptance, interfere with performance. The personal domain opens you up to a whole range of vulnerabilities, all of which have the potential to interfere with your level of performance.

The central decision here comes down to this: should you ignore these dimensions and just do the best you can, or should you actively engage it even though it may initially impair your performance? There is a strong tendency to push the personal out of the way. The decision to grapple with these issues will almost certainly impair performance capacities *initially*. The problem is that the temporary nature of this decline is not part of the unseasoned perspective. Similar to the U-Theory of performance, we find a peak level that is available through submission and the pre-personal domain. Afterwards, we find a noticeable drop as the practitioner begins to grapple with the emergence of his or her sphere of selfhood. This is only a temporary dip as the self system begins to learn how to leverage and perform *with* the sphere of personhood instead of performing while *denying* the emerging sphere of personhood.

As the practitioner learns to bring all of him- or herself into the activity, the fullness of the self can shine into the performance. When this challenging transition has been navigated, a new envelope of performance opens up and one's objective measurable dimensions of performance break through previous limitations. Furthermore, the subjective felt dimensions of performance articulate more joy as the human being evolves.

The personal domain brings with it a shift in response-ability, a new agency that can enact performance. The authority now resides within. While this increases your capacity for performance, the locus of control can fall into the nasty trap of being uncoachable.

Being uncoachable or unteachable means that the sphere of personhood has gone too far in the other direction. The self system wishes to be an island where the only authority and perspective that is welcomed is one's own. Some believe they must do it all on their own, some have been hurt and disappointed by allowing others to control and dictate how they train and perform, while others find incessant flaws in everyone around them to justify their own self-centrism.

Regardless what the reasons are that support this over-insulated self system, invariably what they miss is the relational dimension and how this can be responsibly leveraged for self-refinement and performance improvement. While it is appropriate to situationally insulate oneself from the influences of others, a chronic contraction into this place misses the valuable perspectives of others, which are essential if you are genuinely interested in the most refined expressions of performance.

The perspectives that are of most value to you are the ones that are able to see things that you are unable to see yourself. Invariably, all perspectives have dimensions to which they are blind. If you look to the right, you cannot see what is on your left. All perspectives are inherently limited.

The two types of limitations that are of most use for us are the *Unseen Emergent* and the *Unseen Shadow*. The Unseen Emergent is the part of yourself that has yet to develop and evolve. These dimensions are part of your emergent unconscious. You do not know them and cannot see them because they have yet to show up in your body-mind's unfolding.

One of the beautiful dimensions of humanity is that there are always people ahead of you leading the way. Dimensions of what is latent within your Unseen Emergent are likely an embodied actuality to some degree in someone else. As a result, these individuals can see aspects of you that have yet to emerge and can help you grow into these aspects.

This is not to say that these special individuals in your life know you better than you know yourself. They just know more evolved dimensions of the territory of humanity within themselves, and therefore they can see possibilities within other people. While their perspective transcends your own, they do not know the specific particularities within which you will enact your emerging novelty. Only you can see, feel and experience the inspired emergence that you are in the process of Becoming.

Our personal perspectives are not only intrinsically limited but also attempt to reject, deny and disown facets of ourselves. Most commonly these parts of ourselves inhabit a territory that is painful, vulnerable or uncomfortable on some level. This is the Unseen Shadow, and includes things that others know about you that you manage to remain ignorant of. These are dimensions of yourself that you effectively hide from yourself and, with varying effectiveness, the people around you. These can range from self-sabotage to sets of competing commitments inherent in the unconscious diversion of valuable energy away from your conscious aspirations.

Exposing yourself to a multiplicity of perspectives enables you to see, and thus resolve, more of your Unseen Shadow. As such, it is important for you to keep your self system open to feedback and authentic exchange.

The Problem of Possession

At the heart of the personal domain we find one singular trap that inhibits the further unfolding, expanding and free articulation of your highest levels of performance. Individuals possess qualities that they train, develop, refine and then execute. The trap is the assumption that these qualities belong to them.

This is both good news and bad news. The ability to own, master and manage various dimensions of yourself and your performance discipline is an important step in the process of growing into your greater performance capacities. It is important for the practitioner to assume that at some point they possess the ability to reliably perform at a certain level based on their training. This is indeed part of the process of growing into and performing from the personal domain.

While this is an important *stage* in the development of the human being and the ability to perform, it is not the final destination, and it is not the approach that holds your highest levels of performance.

If you are truly to explore the highest expressions of self, then you must shift *beyond* conventional perspectives and conventional limitations. You must function beyond the personal psychological necessity inherent in possession. Your self system must stretch to your higher developmental unfolding.[31] To do so you must first look directly into a paradox: your conventional self is most drawn to that which it cannot possess. It is that simple. You want, and therefore you cannot have.

The pursuit of possession and ownership is perhaps the greatest invisible virus of which only the most elite are aware; even fewer are immune. As a result, the highest levels of human potential still remain largely untouched.

To gain a better grasp of the problem of possession let us take a brief look at the most basic ingredients of peak performance. The first is the body-mind. We find no peak performance in just the mind, nor do we find true peak performance in only the body. These two dimensions of yourself are not-two. Your body-mind must be trained, well-coached, finely instructed, nourished soundly, supported in an integral fashion and most importantly *well-practiced* if it is going to enact any particular discipline with high degrees of execution. These are the basic prerequisites. Without them, peak expression will remain as potential and nothing more.

The second central element of peak performance is the *moment*. The pinnacle of your performance resides in the marriage of your body-mind with the spontaneous unfolding of the moment. It is with the moment that we find the greatest challenge of possession. Ask yourself this: Do you own the moment? When framed in this light, few in their right minds would say that they possess the present moment. However, perspectives shift when the question is framed differently: Does this moment belong to you? Many people assume, whether consciously or unconsciously, that they do indeed "have this moment." They may say something like, "I have this moment to make something of myself," or, "This is my time to redeem myself."

You do not have this moment, you did not have any previous moment and you will never have a moment. It is important for you to understand this, as your practice, performance and ultimately your ability to work with the territory beyond the personal domain depends on it. The moment *has you*. It is not the other way around.

There have been outstanding innovations in training methodologies, facilities and equipment technologies, coaching strategies and psychological approaches to enhance performance. These are the easier part of the equation in that they all require various types of doing.

When we start to look at the other part of this performance equation, the challenge of Surrendering all of ourselves to the presence of Being, we find challenges that performance programs and their underlying philosophical underpinnings have virtually completely failed to address. And it is on this side of the equation where we find the greatest leaps in performance.

Unfortunately, the entrenched commitment to possession traps practitioners far from discovering their greater potential. As a result, their performance capacities are regulated by harder effort and more work. While they may touch upon what *their* best is, what is lost is the realm of performance that stretches entirely beyond the realm of possession and personhood. While personhood breaks through the limitations of the pre-personal approaches to training, it also brings forth a propensity to hold you back from that which you seek most, the enactment and embodiment of the transcendent.

Chapter Sixteen
The Heart of Performance:
Enacting The Transcendent

The type of Surrender we have been discussing is not a form of "giving up." While your conventional self fears Surrender as a loss of control, it is actually a vehicle through which you can reliably enact the transcendent, or trans-personal.

It is through enacting the transcendent in which the heart of performance is known and the fullness of your Excellence is born. Your conventional self's fear of giving up and thus losing control is more accurately represented as the fear of your own unique Excellence for it is this emergent that your conventional self cannot control. At a fundamental level the personal sphere of functioning and its selfhood is afraid of the fullness of who you really are and what you are genuinely capable of.

The highest reaches of your performance transcend the conventions and functioning of your habituated self. As such it requires great courage to let yourself explore the transcendent territory beyond; for the conventional self, it is akin to dying. The existential condition that supports a compulsive attachment to control and the endless personal investment in the activity of what it is you are doing, have done, or will do must be released.

You may recall from Chapter Thirteen that the primary resistance to Being is the identification with doing. This personal investment in the unending doing activity of life implicitly infuses your activity with habituated preferences. These preferences are not the intrinsic predispositions of the activity of the transcendent unfolding as you, but rather are the work of your conditioned personality. If you are to enact the transcendent and know the heart of performance through your own integrated body-mind, then you must Surrender. You must let go of your intrinsic attachment to doing. You must release your contracted sense of control and merge with the activity of the transcendent moving and unfolding as you.

To step beyond conventional understandings of Surrendering you must merge with the spontaneous activity of the body-mind. Allow your conditioning, training and practice to unfold freely. Release into the witnessing faculty of Being. Here you are no longer enslaved to doing, which, paradoxically, enables you to actually do more.

That which is being Surrendered to is not attached to any activity at all. This is not to say that the transcendent is not invested in the activity and performance of your body-mind. Quite the contrary. The enactment of the transcendent enhances how fully invested and capable you are of enacting your practice. The transcendent's unwavering stance of non-attachment is not to be interpreted as non-investment. The process of attaching restricts how invested you can be. The greater the attachment, the more resistance and struggle your conventional self introduces. With this heightening struggle of attachment comes a potent constriction of the resources you are able to invest in your training.

Again we see that the transcendent adds to the self in ways the conventional self cannot recognize. As the conventional self peers toward the transcendent, what it sees is the dissolution of oneself and the loss of control. Authentic Surrender is not the relinquishment of control but rather transcending the conventional self's compulsive necessity for control. Surrender is the emergence of greater capacities; you are adding to your ability to manage and influence your training, performance and life. As the self transcends the *necessity* for control, you cease to be a separate controlling entity. Your sphere of selfhood envelopes the intrinsic fullness of your body-mind and the unfolding of the ever-present moment.

The greater your body-mind embodies Surrender the more spontaneous and responsive your self's faculties become. Therefore, performance ceases to be an activity to prop up your conventional self's attachments and identification with doing.

Being: Your Doorway to the Transcendent

That which gives birth to novelty most freely is the heart of Being. The seat of Being, the heart of stillness, is Surrender itself. Through Surrender you come to know true devotion and true discipline. You learn how to invest all of you. It is only here that your body-mind can know your true Excellence.

Being rests without boundary as Becoming. This is an important and often overlooked or misunderstood point. While Being quietly transcends all activity and thus rests beyond Becoming (all action of doing, habituated or not), it also quietly inhabits all Becoming without exception. This second point is essential for our discussion of performance. Being and Becoming are not-two, which is why it is only through Being that we find the heart of performance. Being is the only perspectival stance within your body-mind that is non-seeking and non-grasping, and the greatest attunement to what is in the moment will invariably give birth to the most powerful activity in the moment.

Performance that stems from any other seat is intrinsically limited because of various forms of attachment and investment in something else. Your conventional self is built upon struggle; it hopes to recapture a glorious past or focuses on great potential in the future. As a result, performance is subservient to your ego's investment in struggling, not participating, with what is present, resulting in vastly different capacities.

This is not to say that Being eliminates struggle, but it transcends struggle and effortlessly holds your conventional self's compulsive activity. While Being is open, expansive and effortless in nature, this is not to say that there is no effort arising within the open field of Being. Quite the contrary, your training and performance are free to inhabit much higher degrees of effort while resourced by and connected to the infinite expanse of Being. The upper and lower boundaries of your conventional self are shifted (and in some cases temporarily dissolved altogether) opening your body-mind to inhabit the heart of performance.

The Seat of Being and Your Conditioning

Being is fundamentally unconditioned, enabling this transcendent seat to integrate and enact all of your conditioning. It is the space for all Becoming. Therefore, Being actually holds, respects and participates with manifestation's inherent tendency to transcend and include. This is the fulcrum by which we find the intersection between transcendence and performance. When you enact your performance discipline from the seat of Being your conditioning takes on novel capacities.

Consciously joining this intersection between Being and your conditioning brings forth a few major qualities that accentuate your body-mind's capacity for movement. The first is flexibility. Inhabiting the transcendent spaciousness of Being opens the body-mind to enact greater ranges of physical, emotional and mental movement. Awareness becomes much more flexible, and broader perspectives become more available, open and responsive. Emotionally the body-mind expands its ability to conduct greater energy through passion, drive and motivation. Physically the body-mind opens its range of expression whether that be in power, precision and/or endurance. These physical, emotional and mental aspects come together to expand your capacity for adaptive responsiveness.

The second quality is strength. True strength is only born through joining the conditioned body-mind's ability to exert force in the world with the transcendent seat of Being and its intrinsic commitment to transcend and include. True strength has three essential components. The first is your body-mind's conditioning to exert a particular expression of strength and/or power in the world. The second is your body-mind's access to your unconditioned nature, your transcendent seat of Being. The third is the intersection where your conditioning aligns with the natural unfolding of manifestation's inherent movement toward greater transcendence and broader inclusion. It is when you participate with your most basic impulse to evolve from the spaciousness of Being that your true strength is known and articulated.

Strength and power do not serve the conventional self. Strength and power are intimately committed to this basic unfolding and evolution of manifestation. When your body-mind merges with this force, when you Surrender and participate with this underlying current, you stand on a bridge between the unconditioned infinite expanse of Being and the participatory unfolding of Becoming. What is capable from this bridge is distinct from your ego's habituated struggles to possess strength and power for its own limited aims.

The third quality that is brought to fruition through the conscious joining of Being and Becoming is spontaneity. Spontaneity is not "being in the moment." Rather, genuine spontaneity is to inhabit the moment *as* the moment and the intrinsic intelligence of your conditioning. It is through the seat of Being that you are able to freely articulate the innate wisdom of your training and conditioning. This novel synthesis of Being and your conditioning is born spontaneously through your engagement *as* the moment. As a result your integrated body-mind engages as the moment and participates with the evolution and unfolding of the moment in a more refined and attuned way. You are intimate with all that is arising and you spontaneously respond in a way that articulates your Surrender to the greater agency of evolution unfolding as you. The end result is a fluidity and flexibility of your body-mind that inhabits a beauty, power, grace and spontaneity that is entirely inaccessible through mere conditioned effort and hard work through the prism of the habituated self.

This is not to suggest the qualities of strength, flexibility and spontaneity do not emerge without the conscious enactment of Being and Becoming, only that these are naturally arising physical, emotional and mental capacities of your body-mind's conditioning that are accentuated and qualitatively enhanced through the enactment of the open field of Being.

Performance Grooves: The Heart of Performance

What we have been discussing here is referred to as Performance Grooves. Your Performance Groove in any given moment is the inhabitation and enactment of Being and the engagement of your body-mind's unique teleological conditioning. This is your practice and an embodiment of your Excellence, as your unique conditioning is your unique gifts, skills and talents you have cultivated born from your greatest liberation. You are a profound unfolding that inhabits *both* the infinite expanse of Being and the relative conditioning of your body-mind.

Being infinitely invests in the evolution of Becoming, with absolutely no exception. It is through Being's transcendence that you have the capacity to invest in the unfolding emergence of your body-mind's conditioning. This is qualitatively distinct from your conditioned sense of identity investing in itself, perpetuating itself and struggling to exert itself in the world. From the greater perspectives available through Being, you are able to see the uniqueness of your conditioned body-mind. You can begin to see how your strengths, weaknesses, gifts, talents and conditioned strategies intersect with your greater teleological purpose as the transcendent enacting Excellence through your body-mind.

When you merge with and Surrender to the unconditioned presence of Being and the activity of the transcendent, you enact the fullness of your body-mind's groove. Your unique conditioning aligns with manifestation's basic eros. When you join your unique purpose with the limitless rest of Being, your body-mind can know the heart of performance. It is here that you align your conditioning, training, practice and performance with the transcendent's urgent necessity to articulate Excellence as you and through you.

This path is not a luxury. Your life's purpose depends upon this single enactment. This is the path through which you come to know your highest expressions of performance and your emergent Excellence. To fail here is to fail the central part of who you are and why you are here.

Chapter Seventeen
Embodiment and Performance: An Integral Perspective

While performance and productivity are indeed conventional values, the heart of performance stretches far beyond the realm of the conventional self. So while these aims are typically overt values, goals and aspirations of conventional stages of self-development, here we will explore the territory of performance through an integral or post-conventional stage of self-development.

Performance rests as a beacon drawing humanity forward in seen and unseen ways. To unconsciously fall into the conventionally prescribed relationship to performance is to allow this beacon to be converted into a value that solidifies a limited sense of self with constrained functional capacities. The difference between the two is simple: performance either entraps or liberates you. The choice is yours.

The Confrontation with Mortality

We opened this book by looking right into one of the central teachers of life: death. You are going to die. There is nothing you can do to avoid it. As such, there is a limited amount of time for you to live in this form. The more you realize this central truth, the less you protect your conventional self from this realization, the greater your life can become.

Your post-conventional self, your mature integrated self system, is built upon this direct realization. A tangible felt sense of your own mortality is who you are moment to moment. As you grow from your conventional self into your Excellence, death ceases to be merely something that happens to you in the future. In a shift that is welcomed by your unfolding Excellence, you are death. You realize you are that which gives birth to novelty and that which strips down everything such that the transcendent can unfold anew.

Performance is born here. You do not have time (time does not belong to you), you are only offered this present moment. When the illusion that you have time ceases to be a possession, each moment is experienced as more valuable. Therefore, performance becomes an intrinsic articulation of the fullness of who you are.

Without a direct confrontation with death, performance will be locked in the confines of the pre-personal or personal. Your greatness will remain an unknown possibility in a world that needs your Excellence.

The Birth of Purpose

While purpose is first authored in the personal domain, as you step into the territory beyond, you see your purpose is part self-generated and part Surrender. That is to say the heart of who you are is partially your intention and desire, and partially grace and inheritance. It is through this marriage that your performance in training (and life) takes direction and breaks the bonds of your personal attachments.

It is through these perspectives that your efficiency of movement, the power which you possess and the form within your body-mind moves, is perfected. As a result, the frantic pursuit of empty achievements, along with the compulsive attachment to the conventional self, dissolves.

Through this birth of purpose you realize that you are unique. Never again will your particular enactment of life happen. With this realization comes a responsibility, for if you fail to enact your Excellence you have failed manifestation as a whole. The whole Kosmos[32] is laboring for your enacted purpose.

The Integral Nature of Performance

We know that performance is not exclusively a pre-personal nor a personal approach to performance, but must also include the trans-personal enactment of your body-mind. There are four central dimensions that must be navigated skillfully for performance to flower into Excellence. Body-Mind-Moment Training integrates all four of these within its daily discipline such that you continually refine yourself and your performance. It is through repetition that you refine your art. Let us take a close look at each of the dimensions for you to navigate.

1. Highest Stages & Most Stable Foundations

As we have been exploring in the past two chapters, your performance depends upon the stage within which you enact your training. To be stuck in pre-personal expressions of yourself and your performance discipline is to limit your functional capacities to the pre-personal levels of performance. The same applies to the personal dimension of selfhood and performance. Your Excellence, your highest levels of performance, is born from the trans-personal dimension of who you are.

It is your responsibility to enact your self system and training from the highest stages available to you. Your primary tool is Body-Mind-Moment Training. An important dimension to any Integral Practice is cognitive work: the practice of developing your capacity to consider a greater number of perspectives. Ideally your perspectives become more refined and nuanced as you grow. All development starts with the enactment of novel perspectives. Therefore, you have already begun your practice of carving forth novel territory as we have been exploring BMT together.

While enacting the highest stages is essential for you to reveal your Excellence to yourself and the world, so is the enactment of your most stable foundations. Your foundation in strength training is your breath and form. Your foundation for your self system is food, touch, movement, recovery and relationships. If you think of your performance as a building, you want to enact your performance from the top floor, the highest stage with the greatest vantage point. However, if you expend all of your time and attention upon this top floor you will invariably neglect the foundation of your building. It is only a matter of time before the foundation crumbles and the top floor comes crashing down. You must continually return to the fundamentals of yourself, your practice and your training. This strengthens the foundations upon which the highest expressions of your Excellence depend. The higher you develop yourself the greater the demand on your foundation.

2. Creation and Maintenance of Performance States

The heart of performance states is how you are engaged with the unfolding activity of your body-mind within the moment. The more you are engaged the more flexible your performance capacities become. The more distraction your body-mind inhabits, the more rigid and limited your performance capacities.

A state is a temporary shift in functioning of your body-mind. Often states are discussed in terms of consciousness; however, a more accurate perspective on states is to view them as temporary spheres of functioning that inhabit both the mind (consciousness) and the body. Just as a state shifts the functional capacities of your mind, so do states shift the functional capacities of your body.

States allow access to functioning that resides outside your habituated capacities. Traits are enduring functional predispositions inhabited by your body-mind that are an intrinsic part of your self system. Traits are the implicit dimensions of your experience. For example, part of the implicit functioning of your self system is language. You have had access to language since you developed this capacity early in your life. As such, there is no effort, no extra intention or work to use language. It is a functional trait that you possess.

An example of a state would be the complete engagement of your body-mind with the movement during a split squat. As you dive into the immediacy of the sensations, you become the aliveness of the vibrations within your musculature. You hold and enact meticulous form throughout each repetition as you allow energy to circulate through your body-mind. Nothing else exists—there is no thinking about tomorrow, no resistance to the intensity of the moment, only the intrinsic joy of this moment.

As you train in this state, your functional capacity to maintain attunement to your form and your ability to generate power and strength with less effort becomes more refined. Your ability to open your heart to life's unfolding in this split squat is distinct from your habituated way of driving your car. Similarly, your body-mind's functional capacities are different from executing this split squat through the exclusive orientation stage. Your capacity for high levels of movement requires a performance state where your body-mind has access to the integration stage of movement. You can access higher potentials through states that inhabit and integrate your greater developmental and performance unfolding.

So how do you create and maintain performance states? The starting point for the creation of performance states is always intention. Body-Mind-Moment Training starts with one primary intention: to engage wholeheartedly. To create a performance state you must begin with an intention that creates space for a novel relationship with the present moment.

Your intention to engage wholeheartedly sets the stage for the next two steps in creating your performance state. The first is letting go of everything that does not directly connect to the engagement of your performance discipline. Your everyday concerns, stresses, relationships must all be released if you are to have full engagement with your performance discipline in the moment.

Letting go lays the foundation for focus, the central vehicle for your performance states. Once you have a clear intention to engage wholeheartedly and you have let go of all habituated distractions, all that is left is to focus on the process of execution. Within BMT you start with the fundamentals, and from there you build your engagement, state emergence and enactment. Your breath and form always provide the foundation for whatever it is you are doing. Sensation and Being refine the performance state. Mystery and non-duality provide the essential foundations for advanced performance states.

You will find that through the regular practice of BMT and its process of engagement your interior capacity to cultivate focused performance states will improve, even outside of the arena of strength training. Regardless of your performance discipline, BMT will open up new territory for how you create states to support your highest levels of performance.

---

3 Steps for Creating Your Performance States

1. Intention

2. Letting Go

3. Focus

The creation of performance states is only the beginning; you must also maintain your performance states throughout your training. The following three elements are essential for you to manage and maintain your engagement and performance states.

The first is course corrections. In Chapter Thirteen we established that engagement's central obstacle is resistance, and we also established that it is through your various resistances that you can evolve your engagement. It follows then that for you to manage and maintain your performance states you must skillfully manage the various resistances that surface within your practice. Navigating your resistances and thus refining your engagement is course correction.

The second element is refocusing. Though quite simple, this is not necessarily easy to accomplish. As focus is your central vehicle for creating performance states, it is important that you manage your attentional focus upon the right cues. Within BMT you have been encouraged to return to the intention to engage wholeheartedly and then guide your attention to the foundations of your practice. As you reconnect with your breath and form you refocus your body-mind to the appropriate cues, which establishes the groundwork for refined engagement. As a result, higher performance capacities re-emerge.

Again the practice of refocusing within your strength training cultivates your interior capacity to manage the performance states outside of your strength training practice. While the specific surface features of how you refocus may differ within a performance discipline outside of strength training, the defining features you have cut daily through your practice can be leveraged to swiftly manage performance states within other spheres of performance and competition.

The third element is closure, or establishing clear boundaries. The clearer you are about where it is that your performance discipline begins *and* ends, the more freely your body-mind can engage and cultivate highly refined performance states. One of the basic truths of your body-mind and self system is this: You are always working on much more than you know. This is especially the case when you consider refined performance states. Your self system is negotiating and navigating various dimensions of your life and self. All of this is transmuted into the true performance state. One of the reasons that you can successfully let all this go is the implicit understanding that you will return to these dimensions at a later time.

If you have not established a clear boundary of where your practice ends, your self system may introduce parts of your personhood back into the equation prematurely. For example, toward the end of your training you might look at the clock and begin planning the rest of your evening. Perhaps some relational dynamic with your spouse, child or another loved one begins to find its way into your training.[33] These often emerge as a result of not establishing clear boundaries as to when you will actively engage these parts of your life.

---

3 Elements for Maintaining Your Performance States

1. Course Corrections

2. Refocusing

3. Closure

---

3. Attunement and the Management of Relationships

The third domain you must successfully navigate if you are to know your highest levels of performance is relationships. There are two basic types of relationships: intra-personal and inter-personal. You must navigate both skillfully. There are different parts of your self system that must communicate and collaborate if you are going to access your highest levels of performance. Similarly there are relationships with others that you must successfully negotiate if you are to enact your highest levels of performance.

Let us start with the relationships within your self system. Perhaps the most important goal is for you to be highly attuned to the various parts of your self system such that you can meet your core needs. If you fail to remain attuned to the fullness of your self system it is easy for central needs to be neglected. This weakens your foundation and introduces a wide range of problems that will inevitably interfere with performance.

One common symptom of a practitioner who is not sufficiently attuned to their self system is the persistent recurrence of various distractions within the performance discipline. Often the important step of letting go simply does not work. These interruptions within the performance discipline often reflect a lack of attunement with one or more parts of the self system.

What is needed to resolve these performance issues and to unlock higher performance capacities is not necessarily the exclusive focus on the refinement of performance states. While these may be helpful, they miss the underlying causes—the various other parts of one's self system that require tending. Inevitably, parts of you that go without acknowledgment will eventually inhibit and in some cases destroy your performance capacities.

It is important for you to attune yourself to the various complexities of who you are and ensure that your core needs are regularly and consistently being met. Neglect essential needs and you will slay your emerging Excellence. Inevitably central needs will emerge in close proximity to your performance discipline. In these cases it is important that you openly embrace the emergence even though the need may be a distraction.

For example, while preparing for a track meet an athlete gets stuck in self-consciousness. She is not feeling confident, and insecurities about her training and self-worth beyond performing well in her sport are tumbling in her gut and mind. Instead of ignoring these feelings, pushing them aside or distracting herself through music she is wise to spend a brief few minutes attuning to this part of herself. She feels into this insecurity and watches her mind spin out into how ill-prepared she perceives herself to be and to how important performing well in this race is. She feels into the anxiety in her gut even though it is uncomfortable.

Because she is only about twenty minutes away from her race time she does not have the space to work intimately with these parts of herself right now. So, she communicates clearly and articulates what messages she has received and she makes a commitment to herself and these parts of herself that she will attend to her insecurities after the track meet. She will keep this commitment even if she happens to win her race. Additionally she presents a boundary to her insecurity. She affirms the wisdom that may stem from her insecurity but clearly articulates that her insecurity cannot positively help her prior to this race. After openly acknowledging and accepting her insecurities and committing to returning to these challenging parts of herself she shifts her attention back into her task-consciousness which refines the processes needed for her best performance today. While her insecurities are still present they more easily fall into the background as they have been received, accepted and communicated with. As a result her task-oriented consciousness and embodiment stabilizes and her preparation is grounded into embracing the fullness of who she is competing with in today's race. As a result, trust in herself and her capacities to both compete at her best and maintain her inner commitments to herself grows.

Again, if you are able to meet an emergent need, you are encouraged to do so immediately. In most cases, as you are stepping into your performance state, immediate fulfillment of a core need is not possible. Once you have openly acknowledged this need, it is important that you communicate to this part of your self system that you will address it when you are finished with your practice.

There are three elements to integrate into your strategy to successfully negotiate your emergent need. Acknowledgement accomplishes the important function of acceptance, that you hear and understand the self's message. Letting it know you cannot address it in this moment establishes a clear boundary that it is not an appropriate time to act on this emergent need. The final element is a commitment of when the self system will attend to this core need. It is extremely important that you communicate a clear timeline as to when you will address this issue. Even more important is that you live up to your commitment and deliver on your promise to yourself.

The establishment of acceptance, boundaries and commitments, over time, helps the self system let go of various parts so that higher levels of engagement and performance states can be accessed with greater consistency. Ultimately, it is essential that you invest daily in attuning to your self system so you can work with yourself as skillfully as possible.

There are at least four types of interpersonal relationships that can dramatically affect your performance. The first is with a coach. Coaches provide expertise in your performance discipline. It is important for you to review, study, embrace and, when appropriate, challenge the instruction of your coach. Additionally, coaches provide an outside perspective as to how you can improve, what your strengths are and how you can evolve within your performance discipline. The closer you can work with a coach the better, and your capacity to work closely with your coach depends on how skillfully you can manage yourself within this relationship.

For team-based performance disciplines the relationship between teammates is extremely important. Practitioners are encouraged to invest time into learning the strengths and weaknesses of teammates, and it is time well spent if you investigate how best to collaborate with your teammates. Team-based performance disciplines are excellent vehicles for extremely refined performance states as everyone succeeds when the self is Surrendered for the greater good of the team. In the performance states that embrace a genuine Surrender, a greater capacity for performance Excellence emerges.

The relationship with your competitor also contains an important relational dimension that has performance implications. There are two basic kinds of relationships with your competition, and both are essential to your Excellence. In direct competition, you can see an opponent as an object to destroy, humiliate, dominate, etc., and your performance capacities will be inherently limited to these relatively simplistic perspectives. This is because your performance states are directly influenced by the relationship you create and maintain with your competition. In contrast, if you enacted your competition as the vehicle for unlocking your greater Excellence, the sphere of performance capacities would be enhanced when compared to a relational dynamic governed by more conventional dominance-based dynamics. The more nuanced your relationship with your competition, the higher your performance capacities.

As you become more attuned to your competition's range of functioning you can begin to challenge them in new and unseen ways. This means you have a competitive advantage. The greater your competition the faster they will adapt and challenge you in new and unseen ways. This exchange ultimately draws out the emergent Excellence on both sides.

The second kind of a relationship with competition is that which resides outside of the sphere of competition. It is important for you to cultivate relationships with your competition when possible as this provides an important view into the lives, training practices and engagement with their performance discipline. Any one of these holds the possibility for you to shape and expand your own capacities.

The final type of interpersonal relationship is more of a class of relationships. This one fills your life beyond coaching, teammates and competition. These social relationships provide various degrees and types of support and challenge, both of which are required for you to know your Excellence. The central relationships within this social spectrum are family, friends and partners. Each of these relationships provide unique support and introduce unique challenges that call forth a new level of Excellence. It is your responsibility to communicate what it is your self system needs at any given time and to determine whether you feel the present relationship has the capacity to meet you where you are. An integral approach to performance also enacts an attunement with various parts of the self system on an ongoing basis and actively invests in the people critical to the execution of the highest levels of your performance.

4. The Skillful Leveraging of Your Environment

The fourth domain for your consideration is the environment. If you are to know and enact your highest performance capacities it is essential that you learn the art of leveraging your environment to work for you. In any situation you have varying degrees of control over your environment. As such, the more flexible and dynamic you are in leveraging the environment around you the greater the diversity of your performance capacities.

The central principle of leveraging your environment is the skillful use of what is available. If you have a core need and there is no apparent place for this core need to be met, review your environment and assess what is actually available to you. Explore how you can use what is here to fulfill this need. Often by shifting the intention and the way that you approach a part of the environment, you can leverage what is present in your surroundings in dynamic ways that were not initially in your consciousness.

Skillfully using your surroundings to work for you implicitly requires that you know what it is you need, so do not forget to remain attuned to yourself. Leverage your environment to create the right amount of support and challenge that brings forth your highest levels of Excellence.

In summary, your highest levels of performance flower from the fullness of your wholehearted engagement. Your Excellence draws upon the highest stages you can enact through the most solid foundation of your body-mind's functioning. Within this self system, you must create and maintain the most pronounced and refined states throughout your performance window, and your self system must navigate a highly attuned connection with the most critical parts of oneself and the people central to unlocking your greater performance capacities. Your peak performance must be both supported and challenged in the skillful use of your environment. Anything less than this and some part of your Excellence dies.

> **Your Self System *must* Embody:**
>
> 1. The highest stages and most stable developmental foundation
> 2. Access to sustained and refined performance states
> 3. Highly attuned connections with your self system as well as strong relationships with the people critical to the execution of your highest levels of performance
> 4. The skillful leveraging of your environment.

Part Four:
The Territory of Training and Injuries and the Art of Recovery

I completed my last set of leg extensions and suddenly I got lightheaded, so I rested my back up against the wall and slowly slid down into a seated position on the floor. Spontaneously the great path of the 'via negativa' shot through my body-mind. I sat there transfixed as I looked at my legs. I wasn't my legs. I wasn't my body. I wasn't anything I conventionally assumed myself to be but, for whatever reason, I kept looking at my legs. The direct experience was a shattering realization that "I am not this." My body-mind rested upon the ground as something unknown peered through my eyes looking at my legs, but I was something else, something distinctly "other." I was this mysterious vibrant witness. As I sit here and write this I still have no idea where this "I" resides.

Chapter Eighteen
The Domains of Practice

There are four interrelated domains of practice in Body-Mind-Moment Training. These domains are the basic territories of your everyday experience and life. For the sake of simplicity we will first take a tour of each of these domains and then dive into how these domains intersect with BMT and why they are important for the integral nature of your practice.

The four domains are fundamental dimensions of yourself. These irreducible dimensions are, at their center, perspectives. If you neglect or disown any one of these perspectives your self system will experience fragmentation in crippling ways that are often not seen until much damage has been done.

The four perspectives that give rise to the four domains of practice begin with two essential distinctions. The first distinction is the differentiation between interior and exterior (subjective and objective). Right now you have interior dimensions of your experience and exterior dimensions of your experience. The interior dimension is your subjective first-person direct experience. This domain is how you feel right now, what you think, what your mood is, what your dreams are, what your intention is, and so on. These are all parts of your interior as they cannot be measured in an objective, empirical fashion. I cannot know your interiors without talking to you.

The exterior dimension is the third-person perspective of the physical body. This part of you is exterior because it is objective, behavioral and measurable. No one needs to talk to you to know the exterior of you. They can measure your height, weigh you, photograph your body posture, take your blood pressure, draw blood, look at hormone levels and poke and prod you in many ways to come to know your exterior. None of this will directly inform me of your interior, though. While it is possible to know you have elevated cortisol (stress hormone) levels in your blood, a person would know little about how you actually experience stress in your life, how you make sense of this felt experience or if you are even aware of this stress in your life.

Neither dimension is reducible to the other.

The second essential distinction that creates the four domains is the differentiation between individual and collective (singular and plural). While you have an interior and exterior, you also have individual and collective expressions of each.

The collective interior dimension, the domain of intersubjectivity, is the territory of relationships. You have the capacity to engage someone else's interior and they have the capacity to engage yours. Through mutual reciprocity and engagement of interiors we come to know each other. Through this mutual exchange we find a range of relating, from strangers to an intimate partner.

There are also collective objective systems or environments. The state of Colorado, an airport, a gym, a government are all examples of collective exteriors. You have chosen to live in a certain city with a specific set of amenities within your living situation and community. These are inter-objective aspects of your life. A naturalistic observation would reveal all of these facts about you without ever having to say hello. This inter-objective territory is the fourth domain.

The 4 Domains of Practice

	Interior	Exterior
Individual - Singular	**Interior-Individual** Subjective Intentional	**Exterior-Individual** Objective Behavioral
Collective - Plural	**Interior-Collective** InterSubjective Cultural	**Exterior-Collective** InterObjective Social

Perhaps the simplest description of the four domains is this: First-person perspectives are your interior individual "I," second-person perspectives always implicitly involve relationships and are articulated with "you" or "we," and third-person perspectives enact the exterior domains of experience through "it" and "its."

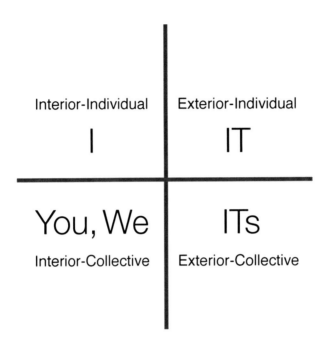

The Four Domains Inside of Body-Mind-Moment Training

These four domains are an intrinsic part of every moment of your life[34]. As such they all contribute important dimensions to this new form of strength training. Let us take a brief tour of how these four domains come to life inside[35] Body-Mind-Moment Training.

1. *The Interior Individual*

Thus far we have spent the majority of our time discussing the interior individual dimension of this practice. For the most part, strength training manuals and the enactment of this performance discipline largely neglect interiors. They wrongly over-identify strength training with the objective behavioral exterior dimensions. The result is a fragmented approach with fragmented results. Our extensive focus upon the interior has been to heal this split, to integrate the divorce between interiors and exteriors and to point out the intrinsic depth you possess and can enact through this discipline. If strength training is only a series of movements you unconsciously move through, you will never glimpse your Excellence; you will only exercise your body, your historical conditioning and reinforce the severance between body and mind, exterior and interior.

2. *The Exterior Individual*

Earlier, in Chapter Fourteen we looked at the process of execution. In doing so we shifted our perspective to the exterior individual. We looked at the two primary dimensions of movement: contraction and extension. We began to explore the developmental progression of execution in which the practitioner is learning how to integrate these two fundamental dimensions of movement. Through this development we find a new flowering of physical capacities for movement and embodiment. We also explored some of the more behavioral dimensions of Body-Mind-Moment Training through the lens of Macro and MicroCycles.

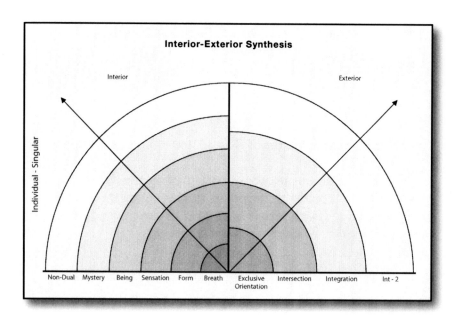

3. *The Interior Collective*

The third domain that must be skillfully navigated for performance to genuinely flower is the management of relationships (the interior collective domain).

BMT requires two basic sets of considerations in the interior collective domain. The first is how you want to maintain the structure of your practice in relationship to other people. Virtually every gym I have ever visited does not have a culture that intentionally and actively supports the deeper pursuits of strength training. While there are a few exceptions, the majority of gyms have cultures that actively accentuate and reinforce fragmented approaches. As a result, much of the social relationships and interactions that unfold within gyms around the world do not facilitate the intentional engagement of your practice. Most interactions that typically arise are distractive.

As such, it is important for you to establish strategies for managing social interactions within your practice such that the process of engagement and execution is not interrupted. There are several strategies that are conducive to minimizing distractive social exchanges. The first is to minimize eye contact since it is an invitation for social engagement. BMT's emphasis upon contraction and extension within the MacroCycles minimizes the opportunities for social distractions because, when you complete the contraction phase of your set, you immediately enter into the extension phase. In between sets (when you have completed both the contraction phase and the extension phase) you have space to accelerate your recovery process.

The second strategy for minimizing distracting social interactions is to stay focused in between sets. You are encouraged to recover between sets in a more private area in your gym.

Finally, if you do find yourself engaged socially you are encouraged to establish clear boundaries regarding your availability to connect.

While there are many parts of gym culture that do not facilitate engagement, one foundational practice that is almost always respected is that you do not talk to the person lifting. While there are always exceptions, the majority of distractive social interactions begin between the conventional contraction sets while people are recovering or making their way from one exercise to the next. Novice personal trainers and inexperienced friends or acquaintances can commonly carry forward conversations into a set, or in some cases throughout large portions of your training. Again, it is important for you to provide clear boundaries to the people who are engaging you.

If you have your own training facilities it is still important that you establish clear boundaries with your family and others living with you as to when you wish to be engaged. Failure to do so often results in conversations that distract and cut off the fundamental thread of engagement with your practice. These relational boundaries are most effective if they begin prior to your training and extend into any reflective process at the end of your training.

Strategies to Manage Social Relationships Within Body-Mind-Moment Training

1. Minimize eye contact
2. Maintain focus between sets as you recover and during transition
3. Establish clear boundaries with others.

The second major consideration is whether you are going to practice BMT alone or with a partner. The majority of my practice and experimentation with BMT is from training alone; however, I see a rich potential for implementing this training methodology with teams and training partners. BMT also has a potential for personal trainers, strength coaches and performance specialists, especially at the highest levels, to provide an entirely new context to guide, train and instruct their clients.

There are several elements to consider to be successful in a training collaboration. The first is to negotiate a clear set of expectations and agreements with your partner. At the least you must mark a transition between your conventional social relationship and your training relationship. These must be two distinct functional relationships or you are likely to be carrying around a distractive relationship from exercise to exercise. I encourage partners to actively commit to one another for defined periods of time: a month, three months or perhaps a year. Keep your commitments reasonable, and when they expire review whether you are going to continue or when you will resume this practice relationship.

Be specific and clear and keep your commitments to yourself and your training partner. This is not simply a friend you like hanging out with. The purpose of your collaboration is to support and challenge each other to engage and refine the execution of your embodied movement. It is up to you and your training partner(s) to figure out how you are best supported and challenged in this process.

You should be mindful of where your training partner is in his or her own process. You want to find someone who is enacting this discipline from a similar stage of engagement and with similar training objectives. If your training objectives are too divergent you will not be enacting the same movements, and thus you will be enacting two distinct training regimens. In these cases both practitioners are better off employing BMT in a solo practice. Developmental differences need to be considered, but no two people are at the exact same place in terms of their engagement and ability to execute. Ideally you want someone who is at the same "center of gravity."

Finally, it is important that your training relationship extends into a reflective process once you have completed your training. Share elements from your individual experiences such as what worked, what did not work, where you excelled and where your central challenges presented themselves. This reflective process is critically important as it can help each learn from the other's practice. It is important for you to provide honest and compassionate feedback about the dynamics of your training relationship.

Foundations for Training Partners Within Body-Mind-Moment Training

1. Clear expectations and agreements
2. Collaborative agreement to facilitate engagement
3. Allow space for sharing and feedback.

---

4. *The Exterior Collective*

The exterior collective dimension is the environment and equipment you have available for your training. Essentially this dimension boils down to facilities, the space, equipment and location(s) that works best for you. Gyms or recreation centers are, at their core, places for growth and transformation. While this may be true, we also find music blaring, televisions lining entire walls with people staring mindlessly at them, etc. You can often find extensive magazine racks on the way to the cardio area as a direct invitation to split the activity of your body from the activity of your mind.

Regardless of these obstacles I recommend you train at a gym for several reasons. To begin, the culture is almost completely unsupportive to BMT's interior dimensions. This is not necessarily a bad dynamic, though. Stepping into an environment that is unsupportive requires that you become much more self-sufficient in managing the interior space that supports your Excellence, establishing boundaries and refining your focus in the face of obstacles. While you may have an adverse reaction to the culture of many gyms, use this as an opportunity to develop and deploy your greater capacities.

While gyms have this cultural obstacle, they also have an array of equipment that simply is not accessible to most individuals for a home gym. Personally I have never walked into a home gym that was better equipped than a public facility. Even the wealthiest individuals with entire rooms dedicated to training simply cannot compete with even a typical small local gym. Your practice will flourish with greater access to more diverse environments to train in. So when considering gyms, the greater the diversity of equipment the greater the range of expression to explore within BMT.

Home gyms are also perfectly compatible with BMT; you are just going to have access to a less diverse environment to train in. The great advantage of the home gym is convenience, which is a huge predictor of training consistency, though the studies done have not considered strength training in the integral context we have been exploring. When this discipline is a central expression of your Integral Practice and connected to the embodiment of your life's purpose in the world, driving forty to fifty minutes every day (twenty to twenty five minutes each way) for an hour of training is different. Missing the practice that adds new dimensions to your life is what becomes difficult.

If you can set up a dedicated space at home, evaluate the adequacy of the space to hold the fullness of your practice. Usually the gym is one of the last pieces to be set up in a home. Subsequently the gym is often the unfinished corner of a basement. This is not recommended. Your practice is a centerpiece of your life. Your home gym is much more effective if it is held in the same regard as a bedroom, office, living room, etc.

Finally, when you are setting up your home gym you need to consider the diversity of equipment so you can enact all of your major movements. I typically break down training into three basic types of movements: push, pull and locomotion. Pushing movements all move resistance away from the spinal column with your upper body, pulling movements move resistance toward the spinal column with your upper body and locomotion engages all functional motions produced by the legs for movement. Your home gym must accommodate all three of these types of movements in a balanced and integrated fashion.

I also recommend you integrate three main sources of resistance in your home gym. The first type is weights. Whether you are dealing with machines or free weights, the medium of resistance is the same. The second type is pneumatic, the type of resistance created through compressed air. Though less common, these machines offer distinct advantages when practitioners are looking to explore the higher reaches of their capacity for performance. The last type is resistance created through various types of bands and bungee cords. These forms of elastic resistance are essential for exploring more diverse ranges of motion, for warming up and rehabilitating injuries and become essential for many forms of ballistic training. Furthermore, many home gyms will integrate some form of cardiovascular training equipment. This is also important for warming up, cooling down, and as a platform for interval and endurance training.

Sweeping the Domains of Practice

In summary, Body-Mind-Moment Training has four domains of practice. Intention and engagement point to the refinement of your individual interior. Execution points to the practice of continually attending to your individual exterior and intimately focusing on the process of executing at your highest levels. Relationships involve working with establishing the right relational boundaries while training. Finally, environment requires that you establish and maintain a chosen space that can support your ongoing practice.

	Interior	Exterior
Individual - Singular	Interior-Individual **Intention** **&** **Engagement**	Exterior-Individual **Execution**
Collective - Plural	Interior-Collective **Relationships**	Exterior-Collective **Environment**

Chapter Nineteen
Practice Beyond Your Training

As explored in Chapter Five, there are two basic ways to look at and understand Integral Practice and how you engage your central faculties. Thus far we have invested most of our time and attention exploring how strength training can engage all of your major faculties in the *immediacy* of the present moment. This again is the heart of Integral Practice. With that said life is by its nature sequential. First you wake up and eat breakfast, then you train before going to work. You spend lunch with a friend before an afternoon presentation. When you return home you help your child do homework and spend time with the family. Before going to bed you may read a book that helps you refine life's various dimensions.

Life naturally unfolds in a sequential fashion. With sequence also comes progress and future results. This chapter explores some of the spheres of practice for your consideration, outside the walls of the gym, that are complimentary to and essential for Body-Mind-Moment Training. The list of technologies and practices that follow can, when employed over time, improve the full engagement of your strength training and refine the Excellence you are able to embody and demonstrate in your life. As such, this chapter outlines some of the conventional benefits of these technologies and practices when applied over time. This list is not meant to be exhaustive or authoritative. Most of the practices presented below are complimentary or supplementary to BMT. These are presented for you to pick and choose at your discretion. The practices that are intrinsically wed to BMT will be identified below.

The Interior Individual Domain

Meditation

While there are thousands of years of commentary on this discipline, one perspective on meditation is that it is a practice that aims to cultivate greater awareness and engagement with the present moment. If I had to recommend only one practice to adopt in conjunction with BMT it would likely be meditation. This inner technology has been shown to improve physical, emotional, mental and spiritual well-being. Meditation has been demonstrated to improve a broad spectrum of measures related to overall quality of life. Here I will list just some of the scientific findings on meditation. To begin, mediation has been shown to increase measures of human development[36] maturity and self-resiliency[37]. Productivity[38] and creativity[39] are improved in addition to increasing levels of social activity[40]. Practitioners benefit from an increased capacity for academic performance[41], improved cognitive flexibility[42] and IQ scores[43] as well as a refined proficiency for perceptual flexibility[44]. Self-sufficiency[45], autonomy[46] and decision-making[47] aptitudes increase along with more developed levels of moral reasoning[48] and greater emotional stability[49]. Meditators also enjoy enhanced neurological efficiency[50] and increased aptitudes for constructive thinking, broad comprehension and cognitive clarity[51] in addition to higher measures of self-actualization[52]. Interestingly, immune system functioning improved along with other key factors such that meditation practitioners used 47 to 73 percent less outpatient medical care facilities compared to their non-meditating counterparts. Similarly meditation practitioners used inpatient medical care facilities 50 to 69 percent less than non-meditators[53]. Meditation also has been shown to impact aging. For example, long-term meditation practitioners in their mid-fifties are on average approximately twelve years younger in terms of biological age[54]. That is to say chronologically a person may be fifty-five, but from a physiological standpoint this fifty-five-year-old is biologically still in his or her early forties.

Meditation has also demonstrated a capacity to reduce unfavorable symptoms. For example, meditation decreases stress[55], anxiety[56], depression[57], anger[58] and emotional numbness[59]. Practitioners with a variety of psychological and psychiatric disorders that invariably disrupt relationships, vocational capacity and overall happiness in life are also benefited by meditation. Anxiety neurosis, obsessive-compulsive neurosis, chronic insomnia and drug and alcohol abuse all have been shown to be positively impacted[60].

The practice of meditation decreases cortisol levels[61], muscle tension[62], heart rate and oxygen consumption[63]. Brain functioning becomes more orderly with increased EEG coherence[64], greater neural plasticity[65] and refined neural integration within the structure of the brain and nervous system[66]. Meditation appears to accelerate the development and evolution of the body-mind in a broad spectrum of key ways. From your brain's neural integrative capacity to the organizational complexity of your self system, meditation appears to help you evolve at an accelerated rate. Therefore, meditation is indispensable in the role of cultivating the unique potential of the human being.

The point is to practice. If possible, find an experienced teacher or instructor who can guide you appropriately. If you cannot, find some literature to guide you. If possible, find a community of practitioners to support your ongoing practice and your unfolding evolution.

Journaling

Journaling can be a practice where you step out of an unconscious pre-reflective immersion in your experience and begin to think about your experience reflectively. This facilitates your conceptual development by helping you integrate a broad range of theoretical constructs into your own lived experience, creating more clarity in your life, and bringing forth greater insight into yourself and your mistakes, obstacles, goals, aspirations and values.

Without the continued refinement of your capacity to step beyond a pre-reflective identification with your experience, adult development is limited. By stepping back from an unconscious immersion with and identification to your direct experience, you rise from one level of experience to a new level. Journaling provides a liberation from being entirely consumed by your habituated responses to the experiences of your life.

Once you have established a strong, consistent journaling practice you may want to integrate a process called phenomenological reflection. Conceptual reflection is excellent for generating insight, clarity and understanding around your recent experiences and where you are headed. The limitation of conceptual reflection is that it has limited value in helping you relate to what is happening right now. Journaling based on phenomenological reflection is a more refined approach because this process looks into what is happening as you are writing. As such, your reflection imposes fewer preconceived concepts and strategies, is more capable of questioning conceptual assumptions and relates to your present experience in a more nuanced way[67].

In this process you shuttle back and forth between writing and touching into your direct experience. This type of journaling is an important bridge between the more conventional approaches to journaling and a meditation practice that brings mindful attention to the present moment.

Shadow Work

Your shadow is the disowned parts of your self system. These parts are the aspects of your life that remain hidden to you and thus remain un-lived. As far as we can tell the shadow appears to be an essential feature of the human condition. Part of our inherent nature is to deny and "dis-own" various dimensions of ourselves. As we grow and evolve, we reintegrate, recapture and embrace more and more of who we are. There are two central insights of importance for you.

First, your shadow is not dormant. Disowning a part of yourself does not make it disappear, it only generates a fabricated boundary as to what belongs to you and what belongs to others; you "disown" what is yours. Unconsciously you often project your disowned parts out into the world. Much that you encounter in other people that disturbs you actually belongs to your own shadow.

When a dimension of you is exiled the shadow can no longer participate in conscious evolution and thus has an inherent gravity to devolve and regress. Thus the shadow, if left untended, often results in varying degrees of what may be called evil. The shadow inflicts much suffering in your life, both for yourself and others.

When the parts of yourself that you do not like are assigned to someone else, the motivation shifts to denying this person in some capacity in your life. That which you are avoiding through disowning will often be governing your life and relationships in hidden and destructive ways.

The inherent danger of the shadow leads us to the second insight: Your shadow is powerful. If left untended your shadow is capable of great harm. This is the bad news of the shadow; we possess the possibility of doing great harm in the world and to ourselves if we are not skillful with our shadows. However, if brought into consciousness your shadow holds tremendous potential to evolve your self system. Your shadow is a beacon to living your full story, a light pointing to your own greater unfolding.

Your true shadow work is to look into your disowned dimensions and to transmute its energy and functioning such that the shadow dimensions of your self can offer their unique gifts that ultimately serve the greater functioning of your self system. Ultimately your shadow is holding keys to your Excellence. These are invitations to tell the larger truth about yourself. You have persistent beacons drawing you forward to embrace and enact more of who you are. Your shadow is lighting a path to your unique greatness.

For example, let us take the athlete who, during the course of her life, training and competition received the message that it is not okay to have weaknesses. As a result, she focuses solely upon her strengths and continually improves them into ever more reliable, persistent and refined capacities. She focuses so completely upon her strengths that from her perspective and understanding she has no weakness. Weaknesses become part of her shadow. As a result, weakness is disowned from her embrace and awareness.

As a result of this denial she sees weaknesses in all of her teammates and competitors where she alone remains the unwavering infallible hero. When she fails in some capacity, implicit in her perspective is the interpretation that it was a result of someone else's actions. She did not fail; someone else did.

So long as weakness resides within her shadow she cuts off embracing parts of herself that can actually facilitate her own growth and improvement. By denying her various forms of weakness she severs off her greater potential as an athlete. As she pushes away and denies weaknesses within herself she diverts vital energy into rejecting parts of herself instead of aligning her fullness with the complete engagement with her sport.

Similarly if a young athlete denies his own capacity to perform he will see the capacity to perform in many or all of his teammates. His own capacity to perform is cut off, denied and rejected. As a result he feels inadequate, uncertain and lacking confidence in practice and in games. In fact, he feels as though he should not play when it is game time. Here our athlete is denying his own capacities for performing at his best. Regardless of what part of the self is severed off from conscious integration (anger, power, love, rage, joy), the same fragmentation of energy results in diminished functioning. This points us to one central consideration: it is wise to integrate a shadow practice into the set of practices that you choose to support your evolution and unfolding Excellence.

Goal Setting

In the 1980s goal setting became understood more clearly by the scientific community as a significant contributor to both high levels of performance and more pronounced levels of motivation in sport. Goal setting has increasingly become part of the implicit and explicit performance culture in sports and beyond ever since.

Goal setting has four functional dimensions[68] that make it powerful and efficient when employed properly:

1. Goals focus your attention.
2. Goals facilitate the mastery of skills.
3. Goals increases the effort put forth.
4. Goals support your persistence in the face of adversity.

Clearly defined goals continually cause you to focus your attention on a task or skill that is necessary to achieve your goal. This periodic and continual refocusing of your attention facilitates greater mastery of skills and performance improvements. Goals increase the effort you put forth into a specific activity because of a higher level of investment in achieving your goal. Effective goals also promote persistence. When you commit to a goal or a set of goals you return to the necessary tasks you might otherwise not focus upon during the course of life's competing demands. Goals facilitate consistent practice and engagement over long periods of time, all of which are requisites for your emergent Excellence. Finally, goals facilitate the development of new learning strategies. Goals provide challenges that frustrate your existing capacities and force you to learn, grow, adapt and evolve.

The most effective goal setting requires an integrative approach, or what's called a multiple goal strategy that employs all three of the major types of goals. The first type of goals are outcome goals. Examples are winning a competition or landing a new job. Generally these goals involve some sort of interpersonal comparison. Performance goals are the second type. These are end products of performance that are relatively independent of the influence of other people or performers. These may be split times, weight loads, completions, accounts landed, etc.—just about any measurement of your personal performance and personal records not directly dependent on an "opponent."

The third and final type are process goals. Process goals are the bedrock of peak performance as they are the most fundamental to the articulation of your Excellence. Most elite performers will tell you that their process goals are the most important to them. Process goals are specific practices exhibited during training and/or in the theater of performance. A runner's focus upon breathing rhythm or running form are examples of process goals. Regardless of what area of your life you are looking to improve, process goals are tools to focus your attention and engagement upon the fundamental elements you must execute to perform at your highest levels.

It is useful to seek an experienced professional or coach who is highly competent in the discipline you seek to grow your performance capacities. Their perspective and experience can help you move forward efficiently with establishing clear effective goals. Here are nine principles to help you set the most efficient and effective goals possible:

1. Make goals specific, measurable and observable.
2. Clearly identify time constraints. Choose a realistic timeline in which you will obtain your goal or set of goals.
3. Use moderately difficult goals. These are superior to goals that are either too easy or extremely difficult.
4. Write down your goals and regularly monitor your progress.
5. Use a mix of process, performance and outcome goals.
6. Leverage short-terms goals to achieve long-term goals.
7. If applicable, set team goals as well as individual goals.
8. Establish all three types of goals (see no. 5 above) for *both* your training and competition.
9. Set goals that are intrinsically meaningful to you. If your heart is not invested in achieving a goal, assess the relevance of using it.

Relaxation Training

Relaxation is an extremely important part of practice life beyond your training for one central reason: Relaxation provides breaks from stress. Stress is an amazingly powerful and potent element in your life. Stress is one of the forces that cause growth and development on all levels and dimensions of who you are. If you do not provide a stress in your training your capacities simply will not develop, but provide too much stress and you will see your capacities rapidly erode. Provide the right stress in the right amounts and you will flourish. If you neglect the need to replenish, you risk physiological and/or psychological collapse. Learning to manage stress is an essential skill. Your body-mind increases its capacity for learning when it is in a relaxed yet alert state.

While meditation is one of the most effective forms of relaxation, there are a couple of other practices that are worth noting for their simplicity and effectiveness. Progressive relaxation involves alternating tensing and releasing your muscles. Typically this is performed by lying down in a comfortable position and (starting with the feet) working your way up the body through the major muscle groups one set at a time. By holding a tight contraction for a few breaths and then releasing with a couple of deep breaths you can quickly provide a strategic break from the stressors of your life. Elite performers can leverage this technique on the fly adjusting their tension and stress levels in a matter of seconds. A large physiological and psychological release can occur or the highly nuanced practitioner can negotiate micro adjustments to facilitate engagement and performance.

Autogenic training is more conceptual in that it involves repeating mental scripts that describe parts of your body as being heavy and warm. For example, I may say, "My right foot is warm and heavy" followed by "My right leg is warm and heavy." Each time I say the script for each body part I breathe deeply and feel into the sensation of my body part being warm and heavy. Similar to progressive relaxation, you start from one part of the body and progressively touch into the warmth and heaviness of each part until you have touched into all the major parts of your body. Autogenic training is typically done two to three times a day and takes about fifteen minutes for each session.

Regardless of what relaxation method you employ, your Excellence depends on the capacity to break the chronic levels of stress that constantly press upon your self system.

Perspectival Flexibility

Cognition is, at its root, your capacity to take perspectives. The more developed and refined your cognitive faculties, the greater your perspectival flexibility. The more stuck you are in a set of beliefs, assumptions or perspectives, the less developed your cognition. As a result you are encouraged to cultivate this core asset through the intentional engagement with novel perspectives. While we have touched upon several major practices that naturally grow your perspectival flexibility (meditation, shadow work, journaling), it is beneficial to have a regular practice of intentionally challenging yourself to inhabit and understand more diversity within your conceptual life. This can be done through reading, research and observation as well as through dialogue and taking up new practices, trying new injunctions in your life and immersing yourself in new places with novel stimuli. The greater the complexity and diversity of perspectives you bring into your body-mind the greater your perspectival flexibility and the faster your cognition will develop and unfold. Adopt an intention to step into the unknown, investigate novelty with curiosity and openness and find greater acceptance for yourself and others. You will find your capacity for attunement with yourself and others increases greatly as your perspectival flexibility evolves and unfolds.

The Exterior Individual Domain

Yoga

The practice of yoga is perhaps the most integrative discipline on the planet. As a result, this rich practice cannot be recommended enough. Yoga is also the oldest unbroken literary tradition with people practicing in this tradition for 5000 to 6000 years. This places yoga as one of the most nuanced and refined systems of human transformation available. To be clear, I am not referencing yoga in its fallen forms. While these exercise classes and their teachers are offering some value to themselves and their students, I recommend yoga in its central aims, processes and purposes. Yoga's core aim is an Integral Practice that cultivates all of the major faculties of the human being such that the practitioner can animate the unique fullness of the practitioner's embodied form from the greatest seat of liberation. If you are to practice the true depth of this tradition I highly encourage you to practice with someone who demonstrates mastery in all eight limbs of yoga.

Breathing & Oxygen

The average adult breathes anywhere between twelve and twenty breaths per minute. That is between 17,000 and 29,000 breaths per day. How you take each breath is important, especially for those of you who are interested in the highest expressions of performance, as this is one of your greatest vehicles for optimizing recovery. The more efficiently you can oxygenate your blood and remove toxins, the greater your energy levels and the faster your recovery. Let us say you rarely fully exhale so that you are always leaving about 20 percent of the air in your lungs that would be best expelled and replaced. Now multiply this by 20,000 over the course of a day, and suddenly a small difference in how you exhale has an exponential effect.

It is often the individuals who have more skillfully recovered who have the greater resources for articulating their Excellence and outperforming their competitors. I encourage you to adopt some form of breath work outside of BMT, as breathing is central to your health, immune system, longevity, brain and nervous system, and as such, your performance. Deepen your breathing and you expand the vibrance and vitality of your life. This is one of the little things that makes a huge difference.

There are a number of breathing practices and technologies available to you. Here are just a few.

a. *Yogic Breathing*—I am not going to go into depth around all of the various techniques and types of breathing within the yogic traditions, but one type involves breathing fully down into perineum, belly and back and then expanding the breath into your sides, and continuing up into your rib cage and chest. You then release the air slowly in the reverse order, fully exhaling. This type of full-body breathing can easily lower the number of breaths you take per minute to around six. Studies have shown that yogic breathing can lower breathing rates[69], increase blood oxygen concentrations[70] and increase lung capacity on exercise tests[71]. For every breath in which you do not optimize your oxygen uptake and maximize the release of carbon dioxide you are actively limiting yourself.

b. A second technology that endurance athletes are known for using is Altitude Training Systems, which simulates training at high altitudes where there is less oxygen available. This type of training forces the body-mind to adapt to lower levels of oxygen while still being able to generate power for high-intensity movement, training and competition. This technology significantly increases your capacity for oxygen uptake and delivery by increasing the number of red blood cells in circulation. When the same training load is then introduced at a lower altitude (with more oxygen) the resulting performance gains can be tremendous. Common benefits include increased efficiency of mitochondria, enhanced physiological power output for increased speed, power, strength and endurance, reduced blood lactate levels at high work loads and accelerated post-training recovery times.

Oxygen tents are also a type of altitude training system that may be useful, although oxygen tents are typically used for sleeping, not training. Here oxygen density is again manipulated to stimulate higher cellular mitochondria density among other advantageous cellular adaptations and wellness benefits.

While placing yourself in oxygen-deprived environments can be advantageous for stimulating physiological adaptations, placing yourself in oxygen-rich environments is one of the most effective practices for accelerating recovery. Hyperbaric chambers come in two types: hard shell and portable.

c. Hyperbaric chambers function by increasing the atmospheric pressure while you are in the chamber and thus increases the oxygen density available to you. The air that you breath at sea level is about 21 percent oxygen and is considered 1 atmosphere absolute (or 1 ATA). A typical portable hyperbaric chamber that compresses air to 1.3 ATA (and does not add any additional oxygen) delivers air that's approximately 26 percent oxygen. While this may not seem like much of a difference, the 5 percent increase in oxygen along with the increased atmospheric pressure virtually saturates the blood cell's capacity to transport oxygen. Furthermore, because of the increase in atmospheric pressure, oxygen transfer by blood plasma is significantly increased. Many professionals agree that even small increases in blood plasma oxygen concentrations can have significant effects upon recovery, health and wellness. Experts working with elite athletes commonly recommend using hyperbaric sessions one time per week on a day you do not train.

It is important to note that portable hyperbaric chambers are extremely safe, with one exception. If oxygen is added, meaning you are not just compressing room air, it is highly recommended that treatments are administered and monitored by a trained professional. Oxygen is extremely powerful and thus high levels of oxygen must be monitored carefully. Too much can do great harm and even cause death.

Binaural Brain State Entrainment

Binaural Brain State Entrainment, often referred to as binaural beats, uses sound delivered separately to each ear to create changes in the functioning of your brain. By introducing slightly different tones or beats to each ear, your brain makes sense of these subtle variations by producing a single subjectively experienced beat or tone.

This may not sound impressive but the frequency-following response your brain employs when you listen to binaural beats does not just occur in the auditory centers of the brain. Your whole brain resonates with the binaural frequency. This whole-brain integration, or hemispheric synchronization, is a powerful shift from the way your brain typically works. Instead of hemispheric competition and fragmentation, this whole-brain resonance is proposed to provide users with a diverse spectrum of benefits.

Perhaps one of the most important dimensions of binaural beats is how your brain can immediately be brought into a specific range of brain-wave frequency. If you wanted to enter into a meditative state of mind, access greater energy levels, induce sleep or improve your focus you can use binaural technology to do so. It is meditation on demand, relaxation on demand, heightened focus on demand.

Hydration

Hydration is a foundational element of your body-mind's healthy functioning. A slight drop in hydration and you will find yourself suffering significant drops in performance[72]. Dehydration increases the amount of toxins and metabolic waste products within your physiology and increases your risk for some cancers[73]. You can also suffer from cognitive slumps[74] and a greater susceptibility to broad range of illnesses. At 5-6 percent loss of water you will most likely become sleepy, conceptually disoriented, dizzy, and experience headaches and nausea, to mention just a few symptoms. Symptoms become more severe as hydration drops further, and most people die if they reach a 15 percent drop in hydration.

Water is an essential ingredient for all biological processes. Approximately 70 percent of your body is made up of water and about 80 percent of your brain is water. Everything from movement, joint functioning, digestion, temperature regulation to intracellular communication requires water. Water transports essential nutrients throughout the body, channels countless biochemicals amongst enzymes within every cell in your body, removes toxins and metabolic waste products, supports your endocrine system, plays a vital role in the structural integrity of your cells and provides the medium through which your DNA's double helixes communicate with one another. This is just the tip of the iceberg. I highly recommend that you adopt some sort of practice of consciously consuming water or other healthy liquids such that you ensure that you get enough.

So how much is enough? The classic answer is eight to ten eight-ounce glasses; however, if training you can double the metabolic demands for water. A doctor, coach or nutritionist can help you assess how much water you need to be consuming on a regular basis. Typically this will involve taking a look at activity level, body weight, caffeine and alcohol consumption, and what altitude and climate you are in.

While I encourage you to speak to an expert, I also encourage you to trust your own experience as a way to adjust and refine the amounts you take in day to day. Take four or five days and track precisely the amounts and times you take in water. Closely track your energy and hunger levels as well as your ability to focus. Blunted energy levels, fuzzy short-term memory as well as a difficulty focusing are often symptoms of not having enough water. Additionally hunger is often a sign of thirst. Trust yourself and stay connected to how you feel throughout the day.

I recommend that you drink small portions of water regularly throughout the day instead of trying to consume large quantities of water one to two times per day. Your body has a ceiling in the amount of water it can assimilate at any given time, so be conscious about having water with you at all times and sip it regularly to optimize hydration.

Second, drink high-quality purified or filtered water. The cleaner the water you drink the more efficient your body-mind will function. Fruit juices and vegetable juices also provide you with additional water with one added benefit: Fruits and vegetables structure water within their cells much like you structure water within your own cells, which can aid in accelerated hydration. Make sure they are 100 percent fruit or vegetable juice, though, and make sure you watch the amount of sugar you are consuming.

Finally, any beverages that contain alcohol or caffeine are going to accelerate dehydration in your body. They do not count toward your fluid intake, and most of the time you will need to drink additional amounts of water to counterbalance the effect of caffeine and alcohol. I recommend minimizing or eliminating their consumption.

Physical Therapy & Performance Training

Injuries are a part of life and training, so part of your practice beyond training will eventually intersect with some form of physical therapy. Once you have received the support and treatment you need you will then integrate your **PT** scripts into your **BMT** to facilitate your recovery. Physical therapy is often something that people attempt to avoid, but there is no sound reason to sidestep treatment. Consciously working with injuries is a part of how you learn more about yourself and how you can continually improve the quality of your life by working with what is most challenging. We will explore this important topic in depth in the following chapter.

On the other end of the spectrum is the domain of performance training. I encourage you to explore performance training periodically with trained professionals with the knowledge and experience that can refine your movement, training and engagement. Part of the practice of **BMT** is to step beyond your current limitations and boundaries. One way this can take shape is to step into some of the best minds and practitioners who can break through your current limitations with novel techniques and strategies that you have never even considered. Performance training is an important adjunct practice that opens up the training diversity that is available to you. Exploring and embodying your Excellence requires some periodic engagement with performance training in which you intensively dive into new challenges to stimulate novel adaptations within your body-mind.

Sleep

You need to pay special attention to protecting and supporting healthy sleep patterns. Sleep impacts your alertness, memory performance, problem-solving skills, neurological and cognitive functioning, cardiovascular health, body-weight regulation, growth-hormone regulation and white blood cell count to name just a few. Furthermore, sleep is an essential ingredient to anyone practicing Body-Mind-Moment Training as many studies indicate a strong correlation between the intensity of activity during the day and the release of growth hormones during sleep.

Most adults require between seven and nine hours of sleep each night for optimal functioning. Cognitive performance decreases with less than six hours of sleep. A regular lack of sleep may double your risk of dying from cardiovascular disease. A lack of sleep also increases irritability and steals a precious window for muscular and neurological adaptation and growth.

If you do not get enough sleep each night a deficit is created. Let us say you average four hours of sleep a night for six days. Essentially, you have a 24 hour sleep deficit, which is the same as if you had gone 24 straight hours without sleep. If we take a snapshot of the functioning of your brain, in terms of cognitive impairment, going 24 hours without sleep is the equivalent to having a blood alcohol level of .1 percent[75]. Implicitly you feel this so you drink caffeinated beverages throughout the day to keep yourself functioning. While this short-term fix helps you in the moment, caffeine temporarily blocks receptors in the brain that regulate sleep, and the cycle is perpetuated.

While a sleep deficit is terrible for your system, oversleeping is also a problem. You need a balance between the challenges and demands you are facing in your waking life and the recovery you need with sleep.
Seven to eight hours of sleep is recommended for most adults. This needs to be a serious commitment. For most people this involves establishing boundaries and respecting the recovery time you need for optimal performance and engagement.

Additionally, for practitioners who are committed to exploring the peaks of their Excellence, I encourage napping. Naps improve your emotional resiliency, mood, memory performance, refine your capacity to focus and give you more access to your higher cognitive functions. Napping also appears to have significant effects upon your heart's health and provides another window for the multifaceted psychological and physiological benefits sleep provides. NASA's Fatigue Counter Measure Program has found that a forty-minute nap improves performance and alertness. The Sleep and Performance Research Center at Washington State University suggests that naps must be limited in their duration to continue to facilitate your waking performance. Much of the literature suggests naps somewhere between twenty and forty-five minutes are the most effective, though I encourage you to explore what works best for your own physiology. This may take you outside of this 20- to 45-minute window.

Be aware of the cultural assumptions and misperceptions around sleep. The corporate culture and medical cultures praise people for functioning on little to no sleep for extended periods of time. This is an extremely foolish and dangerous cultural bias. According to the National Academy of Sciences, medical errors account for nearly 100,000 deaths a year. Many of these deaths are caused, at least in part, by the cognitive deficits implicit in sleep deprivation. While you may confront criticism from peers who fall prey to this foolish mentality, chances are those who are giving you the hardest time are likely suffering from a sleep deficit themselves.

The Interior Collective Domain

Support

Relationships are an essential support system for your life. We are social beings and as such need people in our life supporting our pursuits. I always encourage people to establish relationships that have one central function: support. You want to choose someone you trust and respect, and who has the emotional and psychological availability to support you. This may be a professional, though a close friend is probably a better choice and it is often useful to create a reciprocal supportive relationship for each other.

Be explicit as to the role you are asking them to play. Tell them what you are working on, what your practices are and where you feel you need their support. Articulate as best you can what you anticipate the nature of the support looking like, perhaps to be able to connect on this once a week, or you may request that they simply offer a careful eye to witness where it is you are struggling. This might also take shape as asking for encouragement and motivation to stay the course when you are feeling particularly challenged. Additionally I encourage you to establish clear timelines around this relationship; open-ended commitments end up fizzling out over time. When the time is up you can approach how you want to move forward.

The more attuned you are to yourself and the more you know the territory of your practice the more clear you can be with the relationships you establish to support your journey.

Challenge

Another essential dimension to relationships is the function of challenge. These relational exchanges provide an opportunity for you to step forward in your practice, life and way of being in the world. Challenging relationships pull you forward and draw more of your capacities into greater life and expression. You are encouraged to establish relationships that are explicitly focused upon challenging you in various dimensions of your life. My recommendation is to choose different people than the individual(s) who is going to be providing explicit support for you. While it is possible for a single relationship to provide both, often it is much easier and more effective to explicitly differentiate between these functional relationships. This way the person is not left wondering which role you would like them to play if you have failed to gain clarity around which would be most skillful and useful for you. Again, be as explicit and clear as possible around expectations, what you need, want and are looking for, and of course, provide defined timelines for you both to commit to.

Consultation with Experts

Experts are an indispensable resource for you to draw from, especially when you are adopting new modalities and when you are confronting new dimensions of your practice. They will be able to provide various perspectives, strategies and ways of understanding your experience that are often a result of years of experience and training you simply do not have. Experts have carved grooves that can facilitate your own unfolding so make sure you keep your eyes open for both experts who can support and/or challenge you in new ways and experts who may be of use for you in the future. Start developing a reservoir of experts who can nudge you forward in novel ways.

The Exterior Collective Domain

As we step into the exterior collective domain our focus is going to shift slightly from looking at complimentary practices to essential dimensions of Body-Mind-Moment Training that have not been touched upon thus far.

Training Architecture

Training architecture requires a massive set of considerations determining the training modalities you choose to deploy in your BMT. Your training architecture provides the structure through which you will enact your training. To establish the training architecture that is right for you it is necessary for you to find clarity as to what faculties you want to explicitly focus on refining for a specified period of time. For example, if you want to increase your capacity for progressive acceleration or starting power this will inform the training architecture that follows differently than if you are interested in maximizing strength, expanding your flexibility or recovering full functional range of motion from an injury. Once you establish your central focus, that is, once you have clarified your guiding intention, the exterior dimensions of your practice can begin to take shape and crystalize around this focus in your training.

Your training architecture's duration is best if it is no shorter than three weeks and no longer than four months. Depending on what faculties of your body-mind you are focusing on will largely determine the interval through which your training moves.

Training architecture has three broad forms: structured, spontaneous and integrated. Let us take a brief look at each.

Structured training architectures are suggested for beginners or individuals beginning a new training architecture that is outside their own level of knowledge and competence. Let us suppose you have been strength training for ten years but you have explored only the

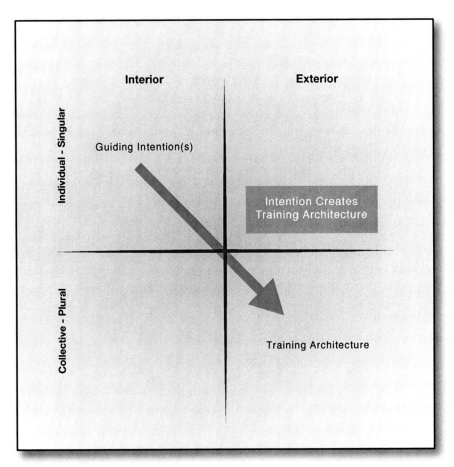

conventional approach to cultivating strength. When your intention shifts and you discover the benefits of training for power you are in need of a bridge. You know how to train for strength but you do not have much experience training for power. Therefore, it is important for you to seek a professional who has expertise with facilitating developmental gains in power. Alternatively you may study some of the key literature on power training. Regardless, you get a structure from someone else's experience and follow their prescription. Your training architecture is structured whenever you are following a prescribed plan.

Spontaneous training architectures are for more advanced practitioners. These still have a clear intention with functional adaptations in mind, however there is a wealth of embodied experience and practice within a particular modality of training. This enables the advanced practitioner to step into their training and follow their own experience moment to moment with greater intimacy. A particular inclination to perform a specific exercise may arise and spontaneously flow into an entirely different way of moving into another exercise. Spontaneous training architectures are extremely rich for exploring the territory of your interior engagement and are vital for the development and evolution of your embodied form. As your self system Surrenders into your emergent capacities for movement, new neurological patterns are laid down and novel capacities unfold spontaneously.

This is entirely different from the commonly seen novices wandering around erratically doing exercises at random. This is pre-structural, meaning there is no structure, framework or direction to their training. The spontaneous training architecture is post-structural, meaning it transcends and includes the structural dimensions of training architecture. You will see that the spontaneous training architecture embodies great degrees of structure, direction and precision; however, there is also a freedom within their movement and how their training unfolds.

The integrated training architecture is for highly refined practitioners who have spent many years refining their structured approaches to their training aims. These appear to the beginner's eye to be no different than a structured training architecture, but to a more nuanced practitioner the structure of the training can be seen as embracing a fluid, spacious spontaneity, where the structure and the spontaneity are not two separate modalities.

Weekly Structure

Your weekly structure is an expression of your training architecture and is also an expression of your commitment to the vehicle of your practice. Simply put, your weekly structure outlines what days you are training and for how long. You will also be identifying what days are going to be used to optimize recovery from the week's demands on your body-mind. Some practitioners may be training only two days a week while other practitioners may be training six. Your structure is your weekly commitment to practice and a way to refine the vehicle within which you will grow and develop your self system and practice.

Fiscal Integration

The final external collective dimension to your BMT is fiscal integration. Often people do not integrate their practice into their economic livelihood. This is one problem of non-integrative disciplines that fracture the territory of your self system and life, and as a result are less effective.

To integrate your economic life into your practice requires you to set up a second bank account or some other form of retainer in which you will be paying yourself for your practice. I know this sounds strange at first, however, this is a fundamental dimension that is often extremely helpful for facilitating an ongoing practice. Once you have your practice retainer set up you need to establish an economic value for the time, energy and effort that you put into your practice.

I encourage you to establish a per-day training value. The majority of practitioners will engage with their BMT one time per day, so a daily training value is useful. If you are frequently training more than one time per day I encourage you to establish a per-session training value. The value needs to be economically feasible for you as you will be paying your practice retainer for each training session you complete. Your training session may be valued at $5, $50 or $500 dollars per session depending on how valuable your training is to you and what is feasible. You can pay yourself once a week, after each training session, once every two weeks, etc. Regardless, it is important that you pay yourself for each training session completed. Missed training sessions are not economically compensated for. If your training sessions are worth $25 dollars and you missed three training sessions last month, you and your practice retainer lost $75.

Over time your practice retainer will grow in value. This fiscal reservoir is to be used to support, augment and grow your training and practice. The sole purpose of this reservoir is to be reinvested into your practice. The fiscal integration is not to be used for any other means of economic exchange outside of reinvesting in your practice. This can take the shape of new equipment, consultations with experts, practice retreats, specific sport intensive camps, massage, books and other media to expand your knowledge base, and so on. Regardless of what it is you decide to spend your resources on, make sure these economic exchanges connect back to your central guiding intentions and training goals.

Conclusion

In conclusion, we have toured some of the complimentary disciplines that reside outside of the walls of your BMT as well as some new essential dimensions. As you can see there is a vast territory for practice and many considerations to explore. Again, while we have swept through the four domains of practice outside of BMT, the list of technologies and practices covered are by no means exhaustive. Regardless of what practices you do adopt and which ones do not fit your life, I encourage you to continue to pick up practices, disciplines and technologies beyond BMT that can support, challenge and ultimately facilitate your evolving Excellence.

Overview

	Interior	**Exterior**
Individual - Singular	Meditation Journaling Shadow Work Goal Setting Relaxation Training Perspectival Flexibility	Yoga Breathing & Oxygen Brain State Entrainment Hydration Nutrition PT & Performance Training Sleep
Collective - Plural	Support Challenge Consultation w/ Experts	Training Architecture Weekly Structure Fiscal Integration

Chapter Twenty
Working With Injuries

Injuries are a fundamental part of your practice life. There simply is no such thing as a committed practice or a life without injury. That said, what *is* an injury within the context of Integral Practice? What is the basic nature of injuries? How are you to work with injuries within your Body-Mind-Moment Training?

An injury in the broadest sense of the word is a kind of pathological disorganization within your body-mind. At the root of an injury is a cause, an event, that has in some capacity disrupted your body-mind's natural or optimal functional organization. Typically, injuries in training are most often referring to physical problems: tendonitis, a torn muscle, a broken bone, etc. However, physical injuries are not the only form.

From a more integrative perspective, pathological disorganization arises within your body-mind, and in this broader context is always both physiological and psychological. Often an injury to one dimension results in some form of disorganization in both dimensions as they are interrelated.

For example, from a physiological standpoint you may receive an injury as you get hit playing a contact sport. This injury's principle domain is within the body; however, a secondary disorganization has been introduced to the mind. In this case, a sense of mistrust and anxiety. Self-doubt consolidates into a contraction with the body-mind that disrupts its open functioning beyond the physiological injury.

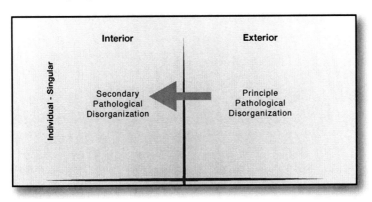

217

Let us take a look at an injury where the principle disorganization is within the interior. Here we may find emotional assaults, violations of personal boundaries, breaks in trust, and/or verbal attacks aimed at the self that can create pathological disorganization. This is often referred to as psychopathology. In this case the exterior (the body) holds the secondary disorganization. For example, an athlete who has spent four years training and performing with a coach who does not trust the athlete's ability to perform under pressure will have significant influence upon the overall functioning of this athlete. As pressure mounts the coach intervenes excessively, sometimes with an underlying sense of anxiety around winning. Year after year this conditioning is reinforced. Our developing athlete now has consolidated excessively rigid neuromuscular patterns that inhibit performance. The injury in this case is a mistrust the athlete has in his or her own capacity. An overly sensitive nervous system has been reinforced that generates excessive physiological stress, especially in the face of pressure. Much of this only undermines the athlete's ability to perform under pressure. Body and mind are intimately connected.

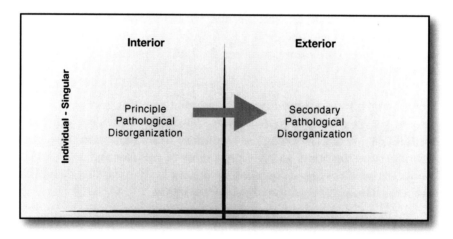

Central Aims of Integral Practice

What is an injury in the context of Integral Practice? Let us take a quick glance at Integral Practice's central aims. One central thrust of Integral Practice, and thus your training and practice of BMT, is to continually expand your awareness so that you know with increasing depth and clarity the fundamental freedom that is intrinsic to your nature. The second central thrust is to cultivate and refine your ability to inhabit your life—how fully you can cultivate and articulate your life in all its dimensions? BMT is committed to the fullness of manifestation, which is why you exercise, train or engage all of the major dimensions of who you are. This expands the fullness and quality of inhabitation you bring to your training and life. If a practice leaves out either dimension it cannot be considered Integral.

Pathological disorganization intrinsically calls forth focused and nuanced awareness into that which has been disrupted. Thus, injuries are a call to awaken, whether the disorganization is principally to your interior or exterior. You get a clearer picture of who you are and how you are organized.

The intrinsic relationship between injuries and awareness is connected to your Witness. The center of your Witness is the seat of your ever-present impartial awareness that holds all that arises. The jolt of injury, the wave of disruption to your body-mind says "WAKE UP!" Injuries innately cut through your conditioned habituation. When you get injured, the most appropriate first response, from a highly conscious level, would be to bow.

Sometimes when working with an injury you learn how to embody Excellence in a way that simply was not accessible to your body-mind prior to the injury. Regardless of the type and severity of your injuries they all carry this key message: Intimately inhabit and embrace more of your life, now!

The Purpose of Injury

1. To cultivate your freedom or awareness: to wake up
2. To cultivate your fullness or inhabitation: to enact more of your life.

Ego and Injury

Where do you go if you fail to leverage pathological disorganization as a tool to unfold and evolve your liberated awareness and full inhabitation of who you are? Let us begin by exploring how your ego facilitates and supports the skillful negotiation of injuries, and how your egoic conditioning can slip into patterns that hinder the healing process.

Recall from Part One that the fundamental moment-to-moment process of ego is *struggle*. It follows that your ego is going to struggle with your injury. The skillful negotiation of injuries requires that you include the ego's basic process of struggle; however, a strong Integral Practice does not unconsciously fall into the ego's conditioned struggle with your injury.

The good news is that your inherent contraction can be leveraged to align with your ongoing pursuit to articulate your greater fullness and inhabitation of your life. So when you first notice the struggle with an injury that is habitually unfolding, you are not necessarily off course. The bad news is that you are not necessarily on course either.

Your conventional self's basic struggle circles the desire to eradicate your injury and its accompanying symptoms. Your body-mind intrinsically wants to remove the disturbance to your functional capacities so that you can return to your body-mind's optimal organization. This process is natural. The bad news is that this noble intention for healing and structural reintegration often heightens and becomes a fight to rid yourself of the injury.

This battle with an injury can take many different forms. A particularly dangerous form is what appears to be a missing battle altogether. This is often not a result of an unconditioned acceptance but of the complete denial of the pathological disorganization as a whole. This dissociative process turns away from the injury entirely and attempts to go on as if the injury did not exist. This denial places great risk upon your body-mind by supporting a rapid cascading disorganization. It is often useful to leverage skillful feedback from trained professionals or other adept practitioners who have experience working and/or training with you. Often, that which is invisible to you is obvious to the ones around you.

One common strategy for working with the denial of or dissociation from injuries is to investigate that which is consuming much of your energy. You will often find the genesis of the pathological disorganization in the opposing structural integrity of the body or within the opposing psychological dimension of the mind. For example, if the front of your hip is bothering you and consuming a lot of energy and awareness, look to the back of your hip and your gluteus muscles for the genesis of your pathological disorganization. Similarly if you are struggling with the relational dynamic of commitment, that is, you are overly independent and unwilling to commit, it is often useful to investigate your relationship to being dependent.

Once you have accepted the injury, including the central cause of a pathological disorganization, there is new territory for different types of struggles by your ego. Over-identification with the injury results in an attachment to the disorganization. In the case of over-identification the ego begins to define itself through the injury. "I have an injury" becomes "I am damaged." Instead of possessing an injury, I *am* the injury. This rigidifies the pathological disturbance, and because the self is now identified with the disorganization, attempts to heal and resolve the injury are perceived as attacks upon the self. This additional contraction extends the lifespan of the injury and the disruption to your body-mind.

Identification & Injuries

1. Healthy identification: I have an injury.

2. Over identification: I am damaged.

In the case of healthy identification, "I" remain a separate entity from the injury. With over-identification, the sense of self collapses into and fuses with the injury, thus "I" become "damaged."

Another form of struggle is withdrawal, where the injury is overly objectified resulting in resignation in the face of the disorganization. Instead of pragmatic engagement with the injury the individual will often fantasize about what it would be like without the injury, or may continually revisit the way life, training and practice were prior to the injury. These accentuated forms of struggle fuel an avoidance of who you are. Thus, injuries have an ingrained potential to take on some type of chronic disorganization that becomes the normal organization of your body-mind.

Healthy and constructive struggle with an injury involves the skillful resolution of the disorganization, followed by the reestablishment of integrated functioning. The conventional self's struggle provides the implicit agenda for healing. This is your ego's greatest gift for working with injuries. The injury is subtly not accepted and the self moves toward the injury's resolution and integrated healing.

So, there are two essential ingredients for the healthy negotiation of an injury. The dimension that your ego cannot provide is the delicate attunement with the nature of the pathological disorganization itself. Instead of relating to what is, your ego struggles with what is. Thus, attunement from the seat of ego is always distorted and is where your post-conventional self is required. This dimension of your self system has no agenda outside of being present to the direct immediacy of the moment.

We now have the basic scaffolding for what is required for the healthy negotiation of an injury: your ego's intrinsic struggle for integrated healing and your refined attunement with what is. Anything less than this impedes optimal recovery.

The good news is that your body-mind's natural process of struggle starts the healing process. The bad news is, left to its own devices your conventional sense of self will end up reinforcing, consolidating and solidifying the disorganization within your body-mind if this process of struggle is not balanced with the transcendent capacity for intimate attunement with your injury. When you allow yourself to embody both your ego's struggle for healing and your unconditioned attunement with what is, you can skillfully navigate your injury to give birth to your emergent Excellence.

Working with the Envelope

Your refined attunement and your ego's intrinsic striving for integrated healing creates what I call the "Envelope." Your Envelope is the territory between your healthy functioning and where your pathological disorganization begins.

Finding your Envelope is an ongoing process once you begin working with your injury. This process involves feeling into your body-mind's sphere of functioning. How you feel into your injury involves a delicate balance between discovering where your disorganization begins and ends and what the nature of this injury is, and your capacity to attune yourself to the disorganization. It is through the gentle intention to explore and

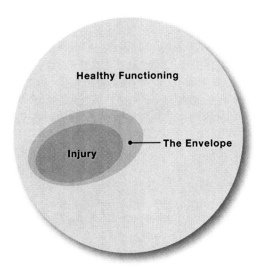

heal coupled with your capacity for refined attunement that you begin to bump up against and participate with your injury. The closer you investigate this territory between your healthy functioning and where your injury resides the more fluid the injury becomes.

This fluidity itself is part of integrated recovery. You begin to nudge up against a part of you that is painful. As you gently press into this part of yourself you feel your physicality constrict. It is here that you stop pushing out and start to feel into what is present. The ego's agenda to eliminate this anxiety is temporarily released and you rest as your liberated body-mind. You watch the images surface, your thoughts weave stories, and you feel into the trauma and damage. As you rest here everything begins to shift and transmute. Your nervous system begins to relax, and suddenly you notice much more spaciousness in your body-mind. Oddly you find yourself within the territory of the injury yet resting in your full presence. Things are okay. They are uncomfortable, but are not the stories you have been telling yourself. You even get a glimpse of how this injured dimension of you actually requires your attunement for healing. As you explore a little further into your vulnerability, your body-mind clenches up, and you once again release the ego's agenda and attune. This is "working your Envelope."

In the moments of attunement it is your sole responsibility to embrace the injury. Your work is simply to be with what is present. It is here that your body-mind metabolizes the injury which then provides feedback for the ongoing process of recovery. You may discover a new way of moving that does not activate your injury, or some other creative emergence may arise on how to work with your injury. Again there is a delicate balance of accepting and attuning to what is and working with what is toward your integrated recovery. Ideally what happens is your body-mind's organization starts to integrate the injury into your larger self system. You become more attuned and fluid with your injury, and over time your integrated healing metabolizes the disorganization and restructures the injury into the greater functional organization of your self system.

While some injuries heal and become fully integrated, others do not and are there for the rest of your life. The trauma, disorganization and disruption to your body-mind becomes a part of you. This is not to suggest that these types of injuries are not workable. This is simply an acknowledgment of your conditioned history, your past and how your present body-mind holds your inheritance. Some injuries become part of the permanent landscape of your body-mind. This is not due to the problem of over-identification but rather the simple truth of your body-mind's experience.

Regardless of whether injuries are resolved or they become a permanent feature of your body-mind, ultimately injuries are to be celebrated as sparks that drive you to engage the fullness of your life from your most essential freedom.

Injuries Within Body-Mind-Moment Training

When you are working with injuries, whether interior or exterior, it is worth exploring whether to avoid directly encountering your disorganization or whether it is appropriate to begin working with your injury's Envelope. A seasoned professional can often provide some guidelines to help you determine what is most appropriate given your unique situation. It is important to note that your BMT is not suited to permanently avoid working with injuries. Training around injuries, when appropriate, is only a temporary strategy to facilitate recovery. Beyond this, your BMT is intended to closely work with the pathological disorganization to facilitate more functional integration with the greater embodiment and liberation of your body-mind.

Engagement with injuries in your training begins as you work with your breath; you begin to explore your Envelope. Subsequently you will discover the appropriate form, both in how you move and where you place your attention within the exercise. Sensation involves a greater attunement with the injury and the surrounding functioning of your body-mind. As your attention inhabits the injury you will gain access to a creative integrated intelligence as to how the breath and movement need to unfold to work with and explore the injury. It is in the novel volitional faculty where the spontaneous and integrated functioning of this stage can metabolize disorganization into functional organization within your body-mind.

The fourth stage of engagement, Being, is actually a prerequisite for genuine attunement. Being is the transcendent dimension of you that attunes to what is. All attunement prior to Being is inherently limited by the activity of the conditioned egoic struggle. The more refined and evolved your engagement is with BMT the more skillful you will be with navigating the territory of your injuries. The less refined your engagement with your practice, the less skillful you will be with navigating your injuries, thus missing an optimal recovery period.

The fifth stage of engagement, Mystery, embodies the heart of this exploration as injuries are a beacon to your emergent fullness and embrace of your life. As you penetrate into Being and embody a novel Surrender into the present, you step fully into not knowing, into the Mystery of both Being and Becoming.

Finally, the sixth stage of engagement, Non-dual, is the seat and suchness of your essential liberation. Your injury is ultimately an invitation to recognize your greatest awareness and unbounded inhabitation of life. Whether you are integrating physical therapy or a psychotherapeutic process within your BMT, the stages of engagement offer you a path for greater skill.

A Note on Working with Professionals

While it is ultimately your responsibility to skillfully leverage your injuries to serve your greater freedom and fullness and to negotiate the territory of your Envelope, I encourage you to consult with trained and experienced professionals who specialize in the type of injury you are working with. Whether this is a doctor, physical therapist, psychologist or counselor, these practitioners are highly trained and experienced and can help facilitate your optimal recovery.

Optimal recovery is not only concerned with the fastest path to healthy functioning but is also invested in using your injury as an opportunity to develop your integrated functioning. Professionals have unique perspectives to offer. Regardless of whether you are focusing on interior or exterior dimensions, the trained specialist can facilitate openings and reintegrations that you could miss entirely. Whenever possible, consult experienced professionals who specialize in your particular form of disorganization.

Chapter Twenty-One
The Art of Recovery

To begin, recovery is the time and space where you prepare from both a physiological and a psychological standpoint. When you have completed a set in training there is always a gap between the set you just finished and the next set you are about to engage. If you are a power athlete, the space between your sets may extend to three minutes or longer. If you are engaged in performance training, the space between your sets could be two fast breaths before you are beginning your next set, or the duration of your recovery may be somewhere in between.

Regardless of what your recovery intervals are, which are largely determined by your training architecture, there is a fine art to optimizing recovery so you are more physiologically and psychologically prepared to move forward in your training. The more you refine your understanding and practice of recovery in training, the more rejuvenated your body-mind is for engagement with the moment and whatever movement is unfolding. The more refined your recovery the higher the level of execution you can articulate. Ultimately, the athlete with the greatest recovery is the athlete with a significant competitive advantage.

While preparation for your body-mind is a core feature of recovery there is an even more significant dimension. While the growth, development and evolution of your body-mind remains at its heart a mystery, we do know that it is in periods of recovery where you are   likely to make dramatic adaptations in response to the demands placed upon it. Often it is in periods of Surrender in which your body-mind is able to structurally adapt and evolve to be able to manage and articulate more of the territory of the self in a more efficient, effective and integrated way[76]. Recovery then is one of the essential platforms through which your Excellence grows, develops and evolves.

We will explore the terrain of recovery as it unfolds within BMT in the four domains of practice we outlined in Chapter Sixteen. Then we will take a tour through these domains as they pertain to your optimized recovery window following training. When you finish this chapter you will have a greater understanding of how you can more skillfully participate with and facilitate this rejuvenation and reorganization process.

Psychological Recovery: Optimizing your Interior

Your optimal psychological recovery has at least three central dimensions. The first aspect of psychological recovery is the intention itself to optimize your recovery. This intention is revisited between each set of your BMT. It is the platform for your body-mind's ongoing adaptations for optimal recovery.

The second dimension of psychological recovery has to do with facilitating the relaxation of your mental focus. Through broadening, relaxing and releasing your mental focus, you refine and accelerate your recovery. Instead of staying in a more habituated mental focus where your mind focuses upon several elements sequentially, you intentionally shift your attention to broaden your mind's lens. This allows your body-mind to relax and thus recover more fully. This pause enhances your mental capacity to focus as you step back into your next set after you have recovered.

Practice: Non-focal Attention

Let go of your eye's habituated tendency to focus upon objects sequentially. Instead fix your gaze three to five feet in front of you and allow your attention to expand and open until you are seeing your entire field of vision without focusing upon any one object. Allow your soft eyes to see everything at once. You will find your eyes habitually falling back into focusing upon singular objects or events that happen in your field of vision. Simply notice when you have fallen out of this broad, open focus and begin to open and expand your attention once again.

The third dimension of interior recovery is psychological space. Optimal recovery requires that you take a psychological break from the stress of your training, engagement and execution. The more intense the training the more precious and important this interior space becomes. If you do not take a break from the stress of your training or generate enough adequate interior space from stress, you will inevitably inhabit lower expressions of engagement, execution and performance. Your body-mind is served when you are able to let go of the training demands as soon as you have completed your set, regardless how short or long your recovery interval is between sets.

This interior space also plays a vital role in your body-mind's capacity to make adaptations. With psychological space, through the dropping of any agenda, you are able to be more open, responsive and flexible in your adaptations for how you recover and how you engage in and execute your training. Periodically you will experience developmental shifts and qualitatively new ways of being and doing in your training. These rich practice moments surface as you grow and evolve in your practice.

Practice: Non-Seeking Space

Resting into your most basic psychological space is broken down into two steps. These steps require refined interior skills. While this section is outlining steps to *do*, fundamentally what is being pointed to is a way of Being that ultimately must be allowed to emerge.

1. *Dropping:* The first step is where your training agenda (and any other agenda present) is let go. Any exclusive focus upon a forward moving direction or agenda is itself a form of stress that inhibits optimal recovery. The challenge that you may already see involves the intersection between holding the intention to optimize recovery and simultaneously letting go of this agenda. An excessive orientation toward optimizing recovery crowds your interior space, which in turn actually inhibits recovery. The intention to optimize recovery must be strong and grounded enough such that you can continue to engage it fully, but you must also hold it lightly such that you can enable psychological space to work for you.

2. *Inhabiting Non-Seeking:* Psychological space is at its heart non-seeking. This state of Being is not headed anywhere, not moving toward anything. As a result, inhabiting this perspective is powerfully rejuvenating. This part of you is wedded to a stillness that is one with the present moment. There are many ways to embody this restorative space. One effective technique is to use voice dialogue and ask to speak to non-seeking space or non-seeking mind. Upon asking permission to connect with this part, you then inhabit and embody this dimension of yourself. You will find that your non-seeking space transcends yet also integrates all seeking activity in its expanse. As you inhabit non-seeking you do not seek to get rid of agendas nor let go of anything because you no longer exclusively identify with these activities. Instead you identify as the non-seeking presence that resides confidently regardless of what is arising within and around you.

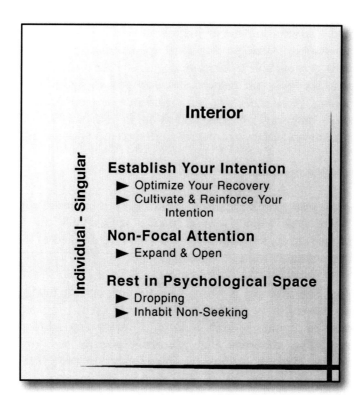

Physiological Recovery: Leveraging your Exterior for Accelerated Recovery

As we look at your individual exterior domain, your physical body, there are two central dynamics to consider for optimal recovery: blood flow and breath. These two processes must be consciously activated if you are to optimize recovery. By supporting these processes your physiology can organize and prepare more appropriately to the demands you are facing in your training.

Practice: Blood-Flow Circulation

Blood Flow is intrinsically facilitated through BMT due to the integrated emphasis upon stretching within each set (recall from Chapter Twelve that a single set includes both the contraction exercise and extension exercise). Stretching increases blood flow and circulation. Once you have completed the stretching dimension of your set and you enter into the gap between your sets, there are two central practices that can accelerate and optimize your blood flow and thus your physiological recovery.

1. *Movement:* Keep yourself moving. The movement is best if it is gentle, relaxed and low in intensity. Walking is excellent because the motion facilitates the circulation of blood. The contraction and release of the leg muscles as you walk is an important mechanism in facilitating blood return from the legs back to your heart. Maintain an upright, relaxed posture and keep moving.

2. *Rest your Hands on your Head:* One of the major objectives when you are optimizing recovery is to maximize the return of blood to your heart. This increases the efficiency through which you can release toxins and circulate more oxygen into your physiology. Resting your hands above your head places more of your body above your heart and thus helps accelerate the return of blood to your heart through gravity. Additionally, raising your arms expands your lung capacity. I do not recommend you keep your hands above your head for your entire recovery period unless you are working with extremely short recovery intervals. Oscillate raising your arms and lowering them to a natural relaxed posture to your side. Practice with different timed intervals. Most commonly you will find ten to fifteen seconds to be sufficient; however, while you are training your legs, this interval may expand, and when your training movements place tremendous loads upon your arms this interval can shorten.

3. *Special Practice—Inversions:* Inversions created by yogic postures or through hanging upside down are not generally recommended without extensive training and practice with them outside of the context of recovery. Inversions provide a number of significant benefits including the flushing of toxins from your organs, increasing metabolic rates and increasing nourishment to your brain. These are not always appropriate given the dramatic changes they produce in directionality of loads and pressures on the spine, as well as the impact they have upon your consciousness.

Practice: Breathing Efficiency

How you breathe plays a central role in the efficiency through which you recover physiologically because of oxygen's central role in energy production. The three dimensions that are most important to focus upon are optimizing your lung capacity, taking full breaths and modulating your nervous system through breathing. Let us take a brief look at each.

1. Optimize Lung Capacity: During the space between your sets you want to maintain an open posture through your spinal column to optimize your lung capacity. Any type of collapsing of your posture impedes the free range of your breathing. Commit to an open posture where your shoulders and chest are open, your belly releases without obstruction and your chin and neck stay open and relaxed.

2. Full Breathing: Immediately upon completing your set you should take three to five full breaths. Take in as much air as you can draw into your lungs and forcefully expel as much air as possible. Remember you are trying to optimize the amount of oxygen you take in with each breath and the amount of toxins you can expel. This means you must consciously work on expanding to take in more air and forcefully exhaling as much air as you can to minimize the amount of stale air that is left in your lungs. Follow your own intelligence on how many of these full breaths you need to take before you move onto the next breathing phase.

3. Modulate your Nervous System: The first two dimensions, optimizing lung capacity and employing full breathing, are universal practices to accelerate recovery. Breathing to modulate your nervous system is an extremely powerful vehicle for accelerated recovery, but it is not fully compatible with some training modalities. Use your best judgement or the advice of a seasoned practitioner or professional to see if this recovery strategy is applicable to your training. Modulating your nervous system through breathing involves mimicking the type of breathing your parasympathetic nervous system uses. All serious training involves the activation of your sympathetic nervous system, the part of you that prepares and engages your body-mind for "fight or flight" responses. Your parasympathetic nervous system cultivates the opposite response and thus brings forward a natural state of rest, relaxation and streamlined recovery. When you are relaxed your breath falls into your belly instead of filling your chest. Your abdominal muscles release, and your diaphragm is allowed to drop down into your belly. This type of breathing places less pressure upon your heart; the movement of your belly breathing massages your vital organs, helping to release more toxins, and facilitates relaxation. In training you will feel the shift when you have gotten past your oxygen deficit; that is, you no longer need fast, heavy breathing to take in oxygen, and there is room for more relaxed breathing. Even when you are breathing down into your belly and activating your parasympathetic nervous system, you still want to be conscious about exhaling more fully to remove stagnant air.

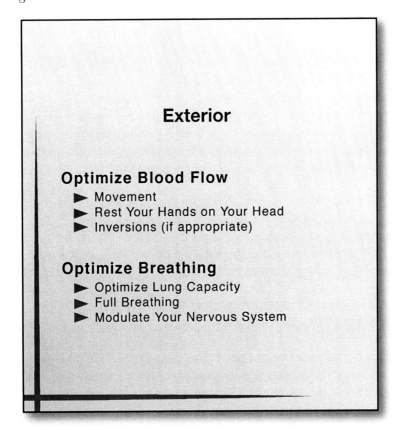

Social Recovery: Refining your Interior through Relationship

Your social persona is invested in and merged with a broad spectrum of social conditionings. Most social interactions often interfere with your optimized recovery as they commonly introduce various layers of expectations, habituated exchanges and ingrained norms. It is important that you avoid distracting social exchanges between sets so your body-mind does not slip into habituated interactions that all too often inhibit your optimal recovery.

One of the central problems of misdirected social exchanges is that they greatly interfere with your capacity to attune to your body-mind. Entering into distracting social exchanges severely limits, and in some cases severs, your capacity to remain finely attuned to yourself. Self-attunement is your foundation for optimizing recovery. As such, you are encouraged to minimize eye contact, provide clear boundaries with others to manage relationships appropriately and stay focused on the physiological and psychological processes that support your optimal recovery.

Training partners must attune to and support not only each other's engagement and execution but also recovery. Partners who fail to adequately address recovery[77] need to be educated on the processes that are most effective for you. Expectations and agreements need to be established. Individuals who fail to hold and respect these agreements should not continue in partnership with you.

Individuals who can see your process of engagement, execution and recovery with greater clarity than you are absolutely indispensable resources. It is possible that by attuning yourself to dynamic relationships with advanced practitioners that you will refine your interior processes of recovery (as well as engagement and execution) at an accelerated rate.

Structural Recovery: Optimizing Recovery through Leveraging your Environment

In Chapter Fifteen we explored how you can skillfully leverage your environment to facilitate the highest levels of performance. Structural recovery also relies on the skillful management of this same territory.

Once again intention plays a central role in the skillful use of the environment you find yourself training in. If you do not maintain the intention to optimize your recovery then you will fail to remain attuned to your self system and miss how your surroundings can be leveraged to

**Minimize Distracting
Social Exchanges**

► Minimize Eye Contact
► Provide Clear Boundaries
► Stay Focused on Processes to
   Optimize Recovery

**Optimize Contact with
Advanced Practitioners**

► Establish Functional Boundaries
► Articulate Expectations &
   Agreements

Collective - Plural

Interior

support you. As you engage and execute sets your body-mind is intrinsically drawn into the form of movement. In contrast as you complete a set your body-mind will naturally orient toward space. That is, you will be drawn to the space between machines, and your body-mind will often seek out open environments. Follow this natural gravity.

Leveraging your environment is in large part the practice of finding the right area where you are able to move without much constraint. You also want to be aware of the habituated ways in which you distract yourself. Bring your full attention to the situations where distracting cues in your environment typically arise, as well as the spaces where these types of interactions occur.

There are some gyms where there is little free space, with an overabundance of distractions and people everywhere. In particularly challenging environments you are encouraged to relate to the smaller places where you can focus and attune to yourself. One simple strategy that has worked for me for years is to place a training towel over my head. I drape the towel so the edge is about even with my eyes. I can see down and slightly ahead but nothing more. This is a simple yet highly effective strategy of leveraging a simple towel to help facilitate self-attunement and recovery amidst an environment that is intrusive to the deeper unfolding of practice.

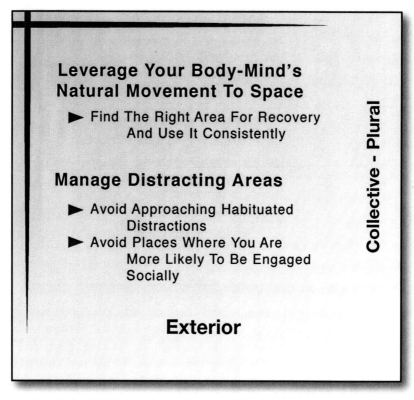

The Relationship to Relaxation and Performance

There is a common premise maintaining that the greater your recovery the higher performance will rise. This is a central orienting premise of some training philosophies and is worthy of some important commentary. To begin, this premise is correct in theory as it pertains, in practice, to the MacroCycles of performance and recovery. The practitioner who recovers most efficiently is the practitioner who articulates the greatest performance (all other dimensions and skills being equal). Theoretically this is sound, and in practice this premise is largely accurate, as long as we are talking about MacroCycles, the days, weeks and/or months, leading up to high levels of training and performance.

Where this premise breaks down is within the MicroCycles of recovery and performance. For example, if we are no longer discussing days between training sessions but rather the space between sets, it is largely *incorrect* to state that the practitioner or athlete who relaxes more completely will be able to articulate the highest levels of performance. This is not the case. As any seasoned practitioner will attest, the highest levels of performance require the right level of looseness, fluidity and relaxation coupled with the appropriate degree of tension and activation. Thus to say, "The deeper the valley, the higher the peak" in this context is false and misguiding to practitioners.

To recover between sets by falling into a pronounced relaxation may not improve your performance, but rather inhibit the fullest articulation of your Excellence. One common trap that commonly emerges when this premise is applied to the space between sets is to get caught in recovery. When you plummet too far into recovery and enter into a state of relaxation that is inappropriate, you may get stuck there. The feeling of recovery feels intrinsically blissful and any activity beyond falling more fully and resting into this relaxation is resisted. If you feel as though you must push yourself out of recovery between sets to then step into the engagement and execution of your training, you have gone too far. Deep relaxation practices are largely employed outside of your BMT, as explored in Chapter Seventeen. However, elements of (not the fullness of) relaxation practices may be used to optimize your recovery between sets within your BMT. Again self-attunement is a central foundation for your recovery between sets, thus you must keenly study and learn how you optimally recover.

Your central objective is to master the fine art of quickly and efficiently releasing psychologically and physiologically to the degree and fashion that works best to support your highest levels of engagement and execution. A common dynamic that is particularly effective is learning to engage deeper psychological states of recovery while using less potent physiological relaxation practices. So your interior explores recovery more fully while your exterior maintains more tension and activation. This is a delicate balance; however, many practitioners performing at their best are able to recover on their interior, which has profound physiological correlates, while at the same time, their exterior physiology is maintaining the appropriate levels of tension for the body-mind to stay in the flow of training and thus allows one to articulate their highest levels of performance. Part of the central challenge of this art is not trying to force yourself into a psychological and physiological state you are not currently in, for this only impedes your recovery. Your optimal recovery necessitates a delicate balance of striving for efficient recovery and the temporary suspension of releasing any agenda so that your body-mind can Surrender, self-attune and recover.

When the art of recovery is skillfully employed through the negotiation of your interior and the management of your exterior coupled with leveraging your environment and relationships, a new territory for engagement and execution opens up. Through intention, self-attunement and practice you will begin to refine the art of recovery. Next let us take a look at some of the key practices for recovery after you have completed your Body-Mind-Moment Training.

Post-Training Recovery: The Art Beyond Body-Mind-Moment Training

The territory just following your training requires some special treatment as this window is a potent vehicle for optimal recovery from a physiological and psychological standpoint. You are encouraged to structurally schedule in the following activities so that you can optimize your recovery between your training sessions. The following recovery practices also apply to competitions and performances. The more consistent you are with these practices, the more efficient and effective your recovery will be.

The recovery window begins when you finish your last set (or alternatively as soon as your competition or performance ends). As soon as you have engaged and executed your last movements the recovery window begins. The window you have to work with is 55 minutes. For professional or olympic athletes, the entire 55 minutes may be used, while individuals placing lesser demands on their training and performance may choose to use only 20 minutes of this recovery window. Regardless of the level you are training at, you are encouraged to leverage all of the following techniques for optimizing your recovery.

1. *Schedule in your Post-Training Recovery:* The first step is a simple pragmatic necessity: If you do not schedule in the time and space for your post-training recovery practices, you are not likely to effectively and

Overview of Recovery Dimensions and Practices
to be Implemented *Within* Body-Mind-Moment Training

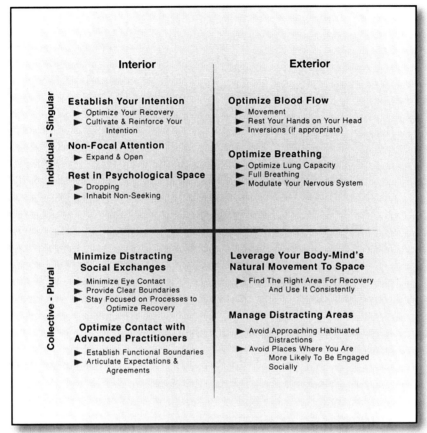

consistently employ these dimensions of practice in your training. If you fail to schedule in this space as a dimension of your practice, your habituated life beyond training will creep in and run over these dimensions of recovery and practice. Some of the dimensions make the difference between recovering in 24-48 hours versus seven to ten days.

2. *Rapid Vascular Flushing:* This potent recovery technique leverages the use of rapid temperature variances to circulate blood throughout your body. By accelerating the rate in which fresh nutrient-rich blood enters your organs and muscular system through applied heat, and facilitating the flushing out of blood carrying toxins and waste products from your vital organs and muscles through cold temperatures, you are able to increase the efficiency of your recovery process dramatically. This

flushing mechanism is most commonly created by submerging yourself in hot water followed by submerging yourself in cold water. The greater the extreme in temperature variance (within reason) the greater the vasoconstriction (narrowing of the blood vessels) and vasodilatation (widening of the blood vessels) and thus the greater the benefits. The ideal scenario involves an ice-tub and a hot-tub right next to each other so the practitioner can submerge in one and then move directly into and submerge in the other. The cold temperature decreases inflammation, pain, muscle spasms and blood pressure on your organs. Additionally the cold temperature slows cellular metabolism, lowers muscle spindle fiber activity and decreases nerve conduction velocity while increasing nerve growth factor, brain-derived neurotropic factor and growth hormone, and improves the function of your immune system. Conversely the hot temperatures are relaxing, facilitate the release of endorphins and reduce stress levels. Skin and muscles loosen due to the increase in blood circulation, and submersion in hot water brings about a reduction in blood pressure while simultaneously increasing your heart rate. The only dimension to rapid vascular flushing that you must look out for is submerging yourself in water that is too cold or too hot. Ice baths are ideally kept around 45-55 degrees Fahrenheit (approximately 7-13 degrees Celsius) while a safe range for hot tubs is 99-104 degrees Fahrenheit (approximately 37-40 degrees Celsius).

a. Your first objective after training is to get into an ice bath or, if this is not available, a cold shower or swimming pool. Your training has produced a significant amount of waste products and toxins that need to be flushed out of your muscles as soon as possible. Your rapid vascular flushing is ideally started with a cold cycle. You can stay in the cold cycle for as short as forty seconds to as long as two to three minutes or longer if directed by a professional. Your hot cycles, either created by a hot tub, steam room, sauna or hot shower, are ideally approximately three minutes in duration.

b. Rapid vascular flushing is most effective when this cycle is repeated at least three times and may be extended to seven to ten cycles based on the intensity of your training.

3. *Personal Space:* While the full 55 minutes need not be reserved entirely for personal space, it is good to establish some boundaries that enable you to privately reflect, learn and integrate whatever has surfaced in

the course of your training. This window immediately following your training is psychologically open and sensitive. After training you will be in an altered state of consciousness, meaning that your interior state is different from your more habituated way of being, relating and acting outside of your training. These altered states can last for varying degrees of time; however, the period of personal space that is tailored to your individual needs and preferences enables two central processes to occur.

a. *Consolidation:* Your personal space enables the shifts and adaptations your body-mind is making to consolidate into your organism's capacity for integrated functioning as you move forward. As you refine, grow and develop, these changes are often subtle and unseen. Occasionally you will have dramatic and rapid shifts in your body-mind's functioning, however the majority of development and refinement within practice happens through subtle emergences and highly nuanced shifts in your body-mind. These emergences are fragile and can be easily lost. Sometimes these shifts go unnoticed as your conscious investment may be in another area of your training and functioning. When you are exclusively focusing upon a specific area of your body-mind's training you are at risk of missing your body-mind's leading edge of development. Another common trap is when your conditioned way of being and acting in your life suddenly snaps back into place after you have completed your training. Without any skillful transition, your habituated ways of functioning can run over and wipe out the subtle emergences that ultimately have much to offer your highest levels of engagement, execution and performance as well as your body-mind's capacity for skillful recovery. Thus a period of open reflection, attunement and integrated learning helps consolidate more of the territory of adaptations your body-mind is inhabiting.

b. *Translation:* Your practice has much to serve the rest of your life, and what is unfolding in the rest of your life has much to offer how you train, practice and perform. Therefore is it most skillful to create a bridge that can help translate what training can offer your life at large and what your life can contribute to your ongoing practice. Your personal space following training serves as this bridge. You are still within your altered state and thus have yet to entirely leave your training, yet you are transitioning back into the demands of life outside of training. Again this period of open reflection, self-attunement and integrated learning facilitates this translation process.

4. Surrender: There is a special reaction when clear intentions and focused striving integrates with Surrender. Whether we are talking about the heart of performance and how to enact the transcendent in your movement, or the subtle work of skillfully negotiating an injury, the acceptance and refined attunement born from Surrendering to Being enables the birth of something much more nuanced and capable of confronting the demands of life, practice and performance. That which gives birth to adaptive novelty most freely and flexibly is the heart of Being itself. Similarly, that which gives birth to the most efficient and restorative recovery is Being itself. Your central road to the establishment and recognition of Being as your body-mind is the path of Surrender. As such, one of the central pillars of your recovery following your training is the practice of Surrender.

a. Just as inhabiting non-seeking space is a central dimension to recovery within your BMT, diving into this same spaciousness is a central process for your optimal post-training recovery. While these practices are similar in nature, the distinction is that you are not briefly touching into this state of Being but, rather, you are plunging and merging with the center of non-seeking without having to hold the body-mind's direction, momentum and flow of training and movement. So inhabiting non-seeking unfolds within the context of training and movement. The practice of Surrender here is referring to a practice of stillness, release and complete relaxation. Psychologically and physiologically you are letting go of and dropping everything.

b. Lay down on your back with your feet shoulder-width apart and arms resting comfortably to your sides. If lying down in this position is uncomfortable for your lower back at any point, roll up a blanket and place it underneath your knees. Alternatively you may use another prop to elevate your knees until you achieve a relaxed posture where your back does not experience any discomfort. The practice of Surrender is simple, though not necessarily easy. Release all tension, stress and holdings physiologically and psychologically ,and rest as non-seeking spaciousness. Do not do anything, just Surrender. For advanced meditation practitioners, you have a choice between your meditation posture or the lying down posture just described. For beginner meditators, you are encouraged to lie down for this practice until your meditation posture has been sufficiently mastered. Your Surrender practice is a minimum of ten minutes; however, given your desire and capacity you can extend this practice longer.

c. In Chapter Twenty, we discussed complimentary disciplines that augment and supplement your BMT. I would like to point to several subsections that may be of service for you as you embark upon a practice of Surrender. The subsection on relaxation training where we explored progressive relaxation and autogenic training are useful strategies to further acclimatize your body-mind to the practice of Surrender. The section on meditation is of particular interest and is again highly recommended, as well as the subsection on yogic breathing. All of these techniques can help walk you to the precipice of the center of relaxation and optimal recovery. Once you have acclimatized, the final step is to simply Surrender and let go.

5. *Recovery Nutrition:* Proper nutrition is absolutely essential for optimal recovery from training. Failing to consume the right combination of nutrients at the right time seriously hampers your capacity for engagement, execution and refined performance. The following are two foundational dimensions of nutrition that require consideration for every training session.

a. *Nutrient Coupling*: Combining carbohydrates and proteins is a proven method in optimizing the performance of your muscular system as well as managing important hormone levels involved in recovery[78]. This combination of nutrients reduces muscle breakdown and muscle damage by improving net protein balance (greater protein synthesis than protein breakdown). Consuming protein and carbohydrates also stimulates insulin (an anabolic hormone) and suppresses cortisol (a catabolic hormone), two hormones actively involved in the recovery process. Cortisol, a major catabolic hormone, responds to the physiological stress of training and increases muscle protein breakdown. Insulin is an anabolic hormone participating in muscular repair and efficient muscle fuel (glycogen) replenishment. Thus, coupling proteins and carbohydrates together results in a greater increase in and preservation of lean body mass and supports the restoration of energy stores required for your optimal recovery. The end result of consuming protein and carbohydrates in the window surrounding training sessions is an increased efficiency in training adaptations as well as increases in capacity for peak performance.

▸ For your training recovery, the most effective forms of nutrients to consume are simple sugars and whey protein. Simple sugars like glucose (or dextrose) are easily absorbed and enter the bloodstream quickly, thus resulting in rapid nutrient uptake by the fatigued muscle tissue. In contrast to simple sugars, complex carbohydrates demand additional energy, drawing more blood into the digestive system, thus reducing the overall amount of water necessary for proper cell function. Sucrose (often labeled as "sugar" on food labels) and maltodextrin (a polysaccharide of glucose units) are also forms of carbohydrate that are easily and quickly digested and absorbed, providing alternatives if pure glucose is not an option. Gatorade powder is a good source of recovery carbohydrate, with the powder form allowing for easy tailoring of your recovery drink. Other drinks that have sucrose or sugar on the label can also serve as immediate sources of recovery carbohydrate. Fructose, the primary source of sugar found in fruit and fruit drinks is not an ideal source of recovery carbohydrate due to its slower absorption rate and potential to trigger gastrointestinal distress. So just be sure to check the percentage of fruit juice in a beverage before considering it for a your recovery matrix. This is the only time that you should be choosing a beverage that is *not* 100 percent natural fruit juice. In terms of protein, whey is one of the most effective for increasing lean muscle mass and aiding in recovery from training. The combination of whey and other milk proteins, along with added sugar makes fat-free chocolate milk a suitable option for a recovery beverage.

b. Nutrient Timing: Optimal performance and recovery require proper nutrition within specific windows around your training. There are two basic options for timing your nutrients. First, when it comes to your optimal physiological recovery from training, you can begin nutritional recovery *prior* to engaging your training and/or performance discipline. A sound body of research indicates that consuming protein and carbohydrates prior to training can help maximize protein accretion and help minimize the physiological stressors associated with training, thus optimizing recovery[79,80,81]. If you choose to time your nutrients prior to training, you are encouraged to consume protein and carbohydrates fifteen to thirty minutes before your session[82]. The second option, and perhaps the most researched dimension for nutritional recovery, is consuming carbohydrates and protein as soon as possible once your training or performance discipline is completed[83,84,85] . Ideally this means you are consuming nutrients within twenty minutes of finishing your training. If you cannot logistically make this happen, it is imperative that you are consuming nutrients within forty minutes of finishing your last set of BMT. The quicker you consume these essential nutrients following your training, the more efficiently they are used by the body-mind for recovery. These are your windows for optimal nutrient utilization. Missing these windows significantly attenuates the efficiency with which you can recover[86].

The movement-specific demands impacting your nutrition can be divided into two basic dimensions. The first is the duration of your training. The length of your training from start to finish informs the amount of nutrients you need to consume for optimal recovery. The second dimension is intensity. Intensity exists on a continuum ranging from low to high, and the degree of intensity you engage and enact impacts both your nutrient coupling and the amount of nutrients you need for optimal recovery. For example, a "short and low" training session will have different nutrition requirements than a "short and high" training session.

c. *Duration:* Training duration can be broken down into three broad categories: short, intermediate and long. Short training sessions are 45 minutes or less. Intermediate training times include any durations where your active movement and training fall between 45 minutes and 90 minutes. Long training intervals are 90 minutes or longer.

d. *Intensity:* Similarly, training intensity can be broken down into three broad categories: low, moderate and high. Low intensity training is principally cardiovascular in nature, meaning that the predominant fuel source supporting your movement (fat) requires oxygen in order to be metabolized. Your heart rate is somewhere around the 50th-65th percentile of its maximum. If you wanted to, you could carry on a conversation throughout your training at this intensity level. Practitioners performing rehabilitation exercises or those just stepping into training after prolonged sabbaticals from embodied movement are typically engaging low-intensity training. High-intensity training involves explosive, ballistic training where your body-mind is exerting high, if not maximal, levels of neurological and muscular recruitment. Both the aerobic and anaerobic energy systems are being challenged and your anaerobic energy system is being stressed to near maximal capacities. Sprinting while attached to bungee cords, explosive jump-training with pneumatic resistance, and maximal RPM intervals on a stationary cycle with variable resistance are but a few examples of high-intensity training. Moderate-intensity training falls between these two extremes where the principle fuel source for movement is coming from your anaerobic energy system. Most conventional approaches to strength training are expressions of moderate-intensity training, even if the training is exploring "point of failure" techniques in a number of sets throughout training. Given the constraints of many forms of strength training involving weights, when incorporating weight lifting into your strength training discipline, you are most likely exploring moderate-intensity training modalities. It is worth noting that training rarely falls cleanly into just one of these categories. For example, it is wise in your warm-up to employ low-intensity movement prior to exploring both moderate and high-level training sessions. After these higher-intensity sessions, a cool-down period allows the body-mind to transition into the recovery process. Ultimately, it is important to determine the predominant center of gravity of your training intensity. Ask yourself where you spend the most amount of time throughout your training. Is it low, moderate or high? This will help facilitate the proper nutritional recovery strategy to support your training and ongoing practice.

Finally, there are two sets of considerations when determining your *personal* nutritional strategy. The first consideration is determining your lean body mass. This piece of information leads to a more tailored nutritional strategy. Determining your lean body mass involves calculating your body fat percentage. Perhaps the most common and most accessible method is caliper measurement. This methodology involves measuring subcutaneous fat with calipers at various standardized measurement areas on the body. Accuracy is dependent upon the skill level of the individual doing the measurements and the quality of the calipers. Bioelectrical impedance analysis (BIA) is another way to establish your body fat percentage. If you use this form of measurement, make sure to use BIA instruments that are used clinically or in nutrition and medical centers, as the technology used varies and thus does the accuracy. For a more robust understanding of your body composition

DEXA is recommended where and when available. DEXA is a dual energy X-ray absorptiometry and is a fast and highly accurate method for understanding your general body composition and much more.

Once you have determined what percentage of your body weight is fat, you can determine your lean body mass. Your lean body mass is composed of your muscles, bones, organs and other tissues that are not fat. For example, let us say a woman is 125 pounds and she has 23 percent body fat. This is roughly 35 pounds of fat. To determine her lean body mass we would subtract her 35 pounds of body fat from her total body weight of 125. The woman in our example has a lean body mass of 90 pounds. Similarly a man 170 pounds who has a body fat of 18 percent has roughly 31 pounds of fat. We then know his lean body mass is 139 pounds.

Determining Your Lean Body Mass

Step 1: **Body Weight × Body Fat Percent = Body Fat by Weight**
Step 2: **Body Weight − Body Fat by Weight = Lean Body Mass**

Female Example:

125 lbs. × .23 = 34.96 lbs. of fat
125 lbs. − 35 = **90 lbs. of Lean Body Mass**

Male Example:

170 lbs. × .18 = 30.6 lbs. of fat
170 lbs. − 31 = **139 lbs. of Lean Body Mass**

Use your lean body mass in the formulas provided in the tables on the following page. These will provide you with the appropriate caloric volumes and ratios of carbohydrates and proteins for your optimal recovery based on your training duration and intensity.

Nutrient Coupling Matrix
Carbohydrate and Protein Formulas

Duration/ Intensity	Low	Moderate	High
Short (45 min or less)	LBM × .08 = grams of Carbs LBM × .10 = grams of protein G of carbs + G of protein = Recovery Matrix	LBM × .18 = grams of carbs LBM × .15 = grams of protein G of carbs + G of protein = Recovery Matrix	LBM × .30 = grams of carbs LBM × .25 = grams of protein G of carbs + G of protein = Recovery Matrix
Intermediate (45-90 min)	LBM × .09 = grams of carbs LBM × .10 = grams of protein G of carbs + G of protein = Recovery Matrix	LBM × .25 = grams of carbs LBM × .20 = grams of protein G of carbs + G of protein = Recovery Matrix	LBM × .40 = grams of carbs LBM × .25 = grams of protein G of carbs + G of protein = Recovery Matrix
Long (90 min & longer)	LBM × .10 = grams of carbs LBM × .15 = grams of protein G of carbs + G of protein = Recovery Matrix	LBM × .35 = grams of carbs LBM × .25 = grams of protein G of carbs + G of protein = Recovery Matrix	LBM × .50 = grams of carbs LBM × .25 = grams of protein G of carbs + G of protein = Recovery Matrix

To give you an example of how the Nutrient Coupling Matrix works, let us say Janet has about 110 pounds of lean body mass and is training at moderate intensity levels for approximately one hour. She would follow the Moderate/Intermediate recovery matrix.

Moderate Intensity / Intermediate Duration

110 lbs. (LBM) × .25 = 27.5 grams of carbs

110 lbs. (LBM) × .20 = 22 grams of protein

28 grams of Carbs + 22 grams of protein
=
Recovery Matrix

Janet knows that her optimal nutritional recovery needs about 28 grams of carbohydrates and 22 grams of protein. To figure out how much food this is from a caloric standpoint she multiplies each figure by 4.

Grams to Calorie Conversion

28 grams of carbs × 4 = 112 calories from carbohydrates

22 grams of protein × 4 = 88 calories from protein

Total Recovery Matrix = 50 grams or 200 calories

Janet now knows that she needs to consume close to 112 calories of carbohydrates and approximately 88 calories of protein and can begin to look for the nutrients and food types to create her tailored 200-calorie recovery matrix. Just as you are encouraged to do, every few months Janet will measure her lean body mass and tailor her recovery matrix accordingly.

The second consideration has to do with your digestive and execution capacity. Depending upon the intensity and duration of your training and your physiological capacity for digestion, you will need to determine your ability to consume pre-training nutrient coupling without negatively impacting your ability to execute and perform. Some people are largely unable to take in nutrients shortly before their training without impairing their ability for execution. If you find that you have a low tolerance for pre-training nutrient coupling, post-training nutrition is imperative. While many find themselves not hungry immediately following training, it is necessary that you consume your nutrients within a twenty-minute window immediately following training.

You now have a sound nutritional foundation for supporting muscular recovery. Based on your specific metabolic needs, coupling the *right* nutrients in the *right* proportions at the *right* time, can optimize your recovery from training.

Remember that, although the window *immediately* around your training is a critical time for precise nutrition, the remaining meals in your day also play a large role in recovery. The main focus for the rest of your day is getting adequate amounts of micronutrients (vitamins and minerals) from fresh (ideal) or frozen sources of fruits and vegetables. Eating a diverse amount of these foods will ensure you consume antioxidants and phytochemicals shown to counteract the inflammation and cellular stress that results from training. Have fun experimenting with different-colored, nutrient-packed fruits in smoothies, adding fat-free greek yogurt for a boost of lean protein. Enjoy huge, colorful salads with walnuts and chopped apples. Or try your own stir fry, an easy way to get a whole day's worth of vegetables in one meal.

Healthy fats are another important nutrient to incorporate. Healthy fats found in canola oil, olive oil, ground flaxseeds, walnuts, and fish oil, are necessary in ensuring proper cell signaling and function. Cook your eggs in olive or canola oil, or try adding ground flaxseeds on top of your oatmeal.

Eating clean throughout the remainder of your day ensures restoration of your body's homeostasis. Remember, there is only one time during the day where refined sugars are appropriate (immediately before or after training). The rest of the day, enjoy *whole*, minimally processed foods that keep your blood sugar stable and your energy high. Consider centering your meals around lean protein: protein smoothie or eggs at breakfast, protein smoothie or greek yogurt at lunch, tuna fish or ground turkey at dinner. Then add generous portions of fresh or frozen fruits and vegetables, followed by a smaller serving of a whole grain (if needed).

Slow down, savor your food, and be grateful for the ability to properly refuel and nourish your body.

If you need help in getting started or coming up with some appropriate meal ideas, look for a local experienced registered dietician (RD).

6. *Establish Supporting Relationships:* You need the time and space to optimize your recovery. Giving yourself this space enables you to get more out of your training with greater efficiency, and this space enables you to enjoy the benefits of consolidation and translation with greater ease. As such, it is often useful to establish relationships that understand, respect and attune to your process of integration and transition. These individuals can provide important bridges for your process of consolidation and translation once you begin to step out of your post-training recovery and begin to enact your life, roles, vocation and relationships beyond your training. Regardless of whether or not you have someone that can understand and attune to your process it is important that the individuals in your life do respect your boundaries around your post-training recovery practices in their fullness. As always provide clear boundaries and be transparent about your needs, preferences and expectations with the individuals who are asking to support your recovery.

As we have seen, recovery is a fine art and an essential dimension both outside of your training as well as within your Body-Mind-Moment Training. The integrative set of practices provided will accelerate and refine your competence for optimal recovery. Whether you are refining your recovery following a set in training or you are optimizing the depth of recovery after you have completed training, this integrative map will help you refine the practice of recovery. You will establish and enjoy being more physiologically and psychologically prepared and you will optimize your body-mind's ability to make creative adaptations in response to the demands you are encountering in your training. And while other practitioners commonly overlook this essential platform or take less integrative approaches to recovery, you will enjoy a uniquely hidden advantage and an expanded capacity for enacting your own Excellence in your training, performance and beyond.

Overview of Recovery Dimensions and Practices
To Be Implemented *After* Body-Mind-Moment Training

	Interior	Exterior
Individual - Singular	**Surrender** ▶ Inhabit Non-Seeking Space ▶ Let Go and Release Everything ▶ 10 Minutes (Minimum) **Engage Personal Space** ▶ Reflect, learn & Integrate ▶ Facilitate Consolidation ▶ Support Translation ▶ Tailor Your Personal Space to Your Individual Needs	**Rapid Vascular Flushing** ▶ 40 seconds to 2-3 minutes COLD ▶ 3 minutes HOT ▶ Repeat Cycles at least 3x **Recovery Nutrition** ▶ Nutrient Coupling ▶ Nutrient Timing (pre or post) ▶ Follow Your Tailored Recovery Matrix ▶ Healthy Eating Throughout The Day
Collective - Plural	**Establishing Supporting Relationships** ▶ Establish Boundaries for Your Personal Space ▶ Generate Support for Your Post-Training Recovery	**Schedule Post-Training Recovery Practices** ▶ Integrate Post-Training Recovery Into Your Training Architeture ▶ Recovery Wondow = 55 minutes

Chapter Twenty-Two
Your Heart's Synthesis

Your life's fullest, most liberated and refined articulation of your unique skills, gifts and talents requires practice. Your emergent Excellence is only revealed through conscious, committed, openhearted, disciplined and integrated practice. Your heart demands your body-mind's unified sacrifice.

Body-Mind-Moment Training holds the capacity to answer life's call for your Excellence. This rich discipline of engagement cuts through your conventional self's habituated deceptions and carves a path into the heart of true happiness. The full articulation of your Excellence rests upon your body-mind's unified capacity to fall in love with your training. Your disciplined practice shapes your emerging capacities that open your heart and engage your life in novel ways beyond your training.

This pioneering approach to training unifies your heartfelt engagement with your refined execution. By synergistically unifying your interior engagement and exterior execution, this discipline transforms the pursuit of performance from a fragmented objectification and denial of personhood to something much more precious. Body-Mind-Moment Training leverages your innate attraction for peak performance as a beacon for your integrated unfolding, and ultimately the unification of your unique body-mind and the transcendent. The heart of your performance is no longer separate from your own spiritual practice and the full embodiment of your radiant Excellence.

Through following your commitment to engage wholeheartedly, by fueling your training with the resistance that surfaces in each moment, you can give all of yourself to your training in service of a precious birth. Through the strength of discipline and the unified application of all your faculties into a single movement you can discover mastery in your own training and life. Through your integrated body-mind you learn how the beacon of performance requires and demands the skillful negotiation of the four domains of practice in your training and life. This attuned skillfulness fosters the art of recovery and draws your full and liberated articulation of your ever-emergent Excellence out into the world.

By shattering your ego's paradoxical relationship with performance, by cutting through your conventional self's habituated and historically conditioned desire to possess and control, the deeper process of engagement and execution comes to life in your Body-Mind-Moment Training. Regardless of whether you are pushing your ego's upper boundaries of intensity through the practice of Surrendered execution or stretching your conventional self's lower boundary as you inhabit the transcendent's non-seeking presence, you are stepping beyond ego. You are enacting the transcendent, which is the embodiment and birth of your Excellence.

This practice has no end. It is your emergent Excellence in every moment that is demanded. No exceptions. The demand is simple, yet the most difficult in practice: Sacrifice yourself fully, without hesitation or attachment. The transcendent's call for you is uncompromising. Your Excellence is desperately needed. Your unrelenting commitment to this moment is a responsibility you cannot ignore.

Our most basic integrity depends upon this integral pursuit of Excellence. Unless you are comfortable with disappointment as you look in the mirror, you must practice wholeheartedly on this path. Strength is your practice to consciously worship the capacity to be in each moment and to align your activity and capacity to do. This is both the celebration of and striving for your Excellence.

Resources

Congratulations, you have taken an impressive journey from your more habituated ways of functioning in training and life to unlocking strength training to yield your larger Excellence in the world. This is no small accomplishment. Take the time to reward yourself with something special to celebrate your newfound freedom to be more and do more in your life. No doubt, you have gained powerful tools to dramatically refashion how you whole heartedly engage with your training and life. You have likely found a tremendous amount of insight into yourself and how you can transform your training. Furthermore, you have discovered new ways to yield next level results as you have traversed through this book. And, books are inherently general. While this book holds years of writing, experimentation and refinement coupled with decades of my own experience training, there is always more to the journey than what can go into a book.

Part of my driving passion and purpose in life is serving people like you. I find myself consumed, often late at night, as I contemplate what people are genuinely struggling with and how novel perspectives, integrative approaches and creative collaborations can help people grow into new ways of functioning in their lives. I work with individuals one-on-one, in courses and in groups from around the world. Some are right here in Boulder Colorado, most are around the United States and spread throughout Europe and Australia. I specialize in helping people leverage the persistent challenges they face in their life to yield their next stages of development. Put simply, I help people get to their next level. If you are wanting to continue to explore your life, training and emergent Excellence in a more personalized way, consider reaching out. Send me an e-mail and we can set up a time to connect to discuss your unique challenges and what tailored next steps may be the most beneficial for you.

You can learn more about me, my offerings as well as contact me through my website:

www.RobMcNamara.com

In the mean time, whole heartedly engage the immediacy of your life. Strengthen your discipline, refine your practice and give the world the gift of your Excellence. Align every facet of your unified body-mind to serve this singular aim and give.

Looking forward to connect with you again soon,

Robert Lundin McNamara

To follow the blog, gain access to media or to learn training tips visit:

www.StrengthtoAwaken.com

Finally, economically supporting the development and implementation of integral practices is an essential feature for furthering adult capacities in today's complex world. Make a tax-deductible charitable donation to support the education, training and advancement of Integral Practices today. To donate and learn more visit:

www.PerformanceIntegral.com

Notes

[1] Evans, W. & Rosenberg, I.H. (1991). Biomarkers: The 10 keys to prolonging vitality. New York: Simon & Schuster.
Strength training has been shown to positively impact all ten of the major bio-markers of aging identified by Western science. The two most important variables determining the quality of life from a Western medical perspective are muscle mass and muscle strength. Strength training is likely one of the most effective forms of movement that can positively impact these two variables.

[2] Dolezal, B.A. & Potteiger, J.A. (1998). Concurrent resistance and endurance training influence basal metabolic rate in nondieting individuals. Journal of Applied Physiology, 85(2), 695-700.

[3] Layne, J.E. & Nelson, M.E. (1999). The effects of progressive resistance training on bone density: A review. Medicine & Science in Sports & Exercise, 31(1), 25-30.

[4] Baechle, T. & Earle, R. (Eds.). (2000). Essentials of Strength Training and Conditioning. Champaign, IL: Human Kinetics.

[5] As cited in Neehall-Davidson, J. (2004). Perfecting Your Private Practice: Suggestions and strategies for psychologists. Victoria, BC, Canada: Trafford Publishing Ltd.

[6] Wilber, K. (1980). The Atman Project: A transpersonal view of human development. Wheaton, IL: Quest Books.
The embedded unconscious is the part of you that is unconscious because of an exclusive identification with a particular psychological structure or process. When you are exclusively identified with something, in this case the struggle with the present moment, you are not able to see it and thus it is unconscious. The embedded unconscious points to the insight that at each stage of development the observing structure or process can not observe its own functioning. In order to be able to see the ego's struggle, that is for it to be an object in awareness, you must differentiate yourself from the habituated functioning of ego. You must develop and inhabit a space that transcends and includes the preceding stage. You must possess the psychological distance from ego to be able to see the functioning of ego. The chapter in hand and the text to follow through this book seeks to help readers gain greater objectivity of the process of their conventional self so to help establish a new developmental seat of functioning in their training (and life).

[7] Foster, C., Hector, L.L., Welsh, R., Schrager, M., Green, M.A. & Snyder, A.C. (1995). Effects of specific verses cross-training on running performance. European Journal of Applied Physiology, 70(1), 367-372.

[8] Zupan, M.F., & P.S. Petosa (1995). Aerobic and resistance cross-training for peak triathlon performance. Strength Conditioning, 17(1), 7-12.

[9] Kohrt, W.M., Morgan, D.W., Bates, B. & Skinner, J.S. (1989). Physiological responses of triathletes to maximal swimming, cycling and running. Medical Science Sports Exercise, 19(1), 51-55.

[10] O'Toole, M.L., Douglas, P.S. & Hiller, W.D.B. (1989). Applied physiology of a triathlon. Sports Medicine, 8(1),201-225.

[11] Murphy, M. (1992). The Future of The Body. New York: Jeremy P. Tarcher/ Putnam.
See chapter 26 entitled Integral Practices.

[12] Leonard, G. & Murphy, M. (1995). The Life We are Given, A long-term program fro realizing the potential of body, mind, heart and soul. New York: Jeremy P. Tarcher/Putnam.

[13] Wilber, K. (2000). Integral Psychology: Consciousness, spirit, psychology, therapy. Boston: Shambhala Publications, Inc..
The term self system is being used here to highlight the complex nature of the self. For example your self system is composed of multiple developmental lines, stages of development and their corresponding traits (both deep and surface structures), transitioning states and typologies to name just a few of your self's major components. It is more accurate to view oneself as a self system of interpenetrating holons (or hole/parts) that interact with one another and with one's collective interior and exterior environment from moment to moment than it is to conceive of oneself as a whole and complete self that interacts in the world as a pool ball bouncing off other discrete whole and complete selves.

[14] Dissolve is being used to describe the quality of the attachment to ego and not the dissolution, breakdown or meltdown of the ego's structure and functioning as in the case of psychotic episodes, some spiritual emergencies and other serious psychological disturbances. The dissolution being discussed is in service of growth as it is the attachment to egoic identification that is breaking down, not the breakdown of healthy egoic regulatory functioning itself.

[15] Cook-Greuter, S.R. (1999). Postautonomous Ego Development: A study of its nature and measurement. Integral Publishers.
While adult developmental theory is a foundation for our discussion, this text is largely an exploration of some of the highest stages of adult development. The enormously difficult and challenging task of formulating and studying these highest levels of maturity has been most elegantly researched by Susan Cook-Greuter. Her life work has established a scientific foundation for the highest stages of identity development and meaning-making that we presently know of through the tool of measuring how people construct meaning through language.

[16] This stage model is a theory based on how human beings tend to develop. The model presented will need to be tested to see if indeed it is an accurate presentation of how people develop in their strength training practice.

[17] Csikszentmihalyi, M. (1990). Flow: The psychology of optimal experience. NY: Harper and Row

[18] For most, Mastery will not even be broached on a consistent basis with 15 to 20 years of disciplined, intentionally guided training. While many will have transitory states of this stage, most of these experiences will go unnoticed by the less mature practitioner. Growing and Thriving states will be recognized more easily; however, they will be less readily available. Mastery states are, ironically, more available yet incredibly difficult to recognize, let alone appreciate and cultivate.

[19] Singh, N.A., Clements, K.M. & Fiatarone, M.A. (1997). A Randomized Controlled Trial of Progressive Resistance Training in Depressed Elders. The Journals of Gerontology Series A: Biological Sciences and Medical Sciences, 52(1), 27-35.
This study concluded that progressive resistance training in depressed elders is an effective antidepressant and that progressive strength training also improved strength, moral and quality of life measures.

[20] Beniamini, Y., Rubenstein, J.J., Zaichkowsky, L.D. & Crim M.C. (1997). Effects of High-Intensity Strength Training on Quality-of-Life Parameters in Cardiac Rehabilitation Patients. American Journal of Cardiology, 80(7), 841-846.
This study found high-intensity strength training improved total mood disturbances, depression/dejection and fatigue/inertia.

[21] Kegan, R. (1994). In Over Our Heads: The mental demands of modern life. Cambridge, MA: Harvard University Press.
Self Authoring is technically not only an emotional faculty but involves at least six core characteristics. The self authoring individual can 1. invent or own their training, 2. self initiate, self correct and self evaluate their training, 3. guide their training with their own values and vision, 4. take responsibility for what happens (both internally and externally) 5. master their training and stand as an authority (as opposed to apprenticing or imitating their training) and 6. see training from from a multiplicity of perspectives as it pertains to themselves as well as others engaged and not engaged in strength training.

[22] Liu-Ambrose, T., Nagamatsu, L.S., Graf, P., Beattie, B.L., Ashe, M.C. & Handy, T.C. (2010). Resistance Training and Executive Functions: A 12-month randomized controlled study. Archives of Internal Medicine, 170(2), 170-178.

[23] Wilber, K. (1995). Sex, Ecology, Spirituality: The spirit of evolution. Boston, MA: Shambhala Publications, Inc.
Development's differentiation phase is a process in which a new capacity has begun to emerge and is integrated into its functioning. As the self system integrates the novel higher-ordered capacities it differentiates itself from being exclusively identified with the preceding self-structure. What was once whole becomes part of a larger more integrative structure.

[24] Frustration is inherent in the differentiation process of growth. There is a natural dissonance or frustration to the self system in any growth process as the sense of self is in transition from one set of self-defining capacities to another more inclusive set of capacities. Without frustrating the existing self system, growth will largely arrest and remain fixed at a particular stage. With the right challenge, frustration, and dissonance, novel emergent qualities can be fostered into a stable home base for the self system to comfortably identify with and function from.

[25] Awareness is at its root timeless, awareness is one of your body-mind's capacities that is transcendent in nature. It is liberation, freedom from suffering, unborn emptiness and so on. Ultimately how Free you are determines how much you can Accept.

[26] Inhabiting at its root is the drive for the fullness of manifestation. Inhabitation is pointing to the drive to engage fully as and with the totality of your body-mind.

[27] Wilber, K. Excerpt C: The Ways We Are In This Together: Intersubjectivity and interobjectivity in the holonic kosmos. Retrieved from http://wilber.shambhala.com/html/books/kosmos/excerptC/intro-1.cfm/
For readers who are steeped in integral theory technically these six stages are an integration of the author's state-stage experiences training coupled with the rigorous study of a number of structure-stage models. A zone 2 investigation of a signifiant sample of BMT practitioners is required to set the foundation for an empirically-based structure-stage model. The stage model present here has been developed from the author's zone 1 exploration and investigation of his own direct experience and study of both state-stage and structure-stage models.

[28] Eventually the first-person inhabitation of your body-mind expands to the first-person inhabitation of your body-mind and the moment, such that your subjective seat is no longer identified exclusively to your body-mind. Your subjective seat, or witnessing and perceiving faculty, transcends and includes the fullness of what is arising in the moment. As such, you are no longer a body-mind in the moment but you are a body-mind and the arising moment.

[29] The term preliminary is being used here to refer to early stages of performance development (and not necessarily time) as disciplines are first adopted. Practitioners can spend many years and in some cases, where performance development has arrested, large sections of training working on preliminary stages of performance development.

[30] Yoga is being used here in reference to the third limb of yoga, asana or the conscious inhabitation of body postures, and is not referencing the full yogic path inclusive of all eight limbs of yoga.

[31] McNamara, R. (2004). Sport Psychology: A developmental-constructive approach (Unpublished Masters Thesis). Naropa University, Boulder Colorado, USA.

Interestingly the discussion of developmental stages of interior development is largely void from virtually every single performance psychology in the world. While many sport and performance psychology orientations study, identify and seek to refine the interior approaches elite athletes and performers have developed, there is a void as to the interior states and stages within which these psychological tools are discovered and implemented. Furthermore, the performance community's apparent blindness to the developmental-constructive nature of performance has left this realm of potential largely untouched. It is one of the central arguments of the author that this interior domain integrated into the rest of an integral approach to performance is in fact one of the greatest sources for performance development.

[32] Wilber, K. (1995). Sex, Ecology, Spirituality: The spirit of evolution. Boston, MA: Shambhala Publications, Inc.

Kosmos is a term created by Wilber to reference all of manifestation. This was principally introduced to counteract the scientific-reductionistic interpretation of the term "cosmos" which is typically used to reference the exterior manifest world. Kosmos acknowledges the interior and exterior dimensions of manifestation.

[33] Body-Mind-Moment Training is perfectly compatible for working with, negotiating, reintegrating and resolving a broad spectrum of issues arising within the practitioner. Many practitioners will require periods of intentional and intense focus upon finding resolution with charged issues that originate outside of strength training through their training and practice. These periods ultimately serve the practitioner's unfolding Excellence, however they are treated as a dimension of the self system that inhibits performance states given the context of the discussion and its aim towards performance. Periods of intentionally working through issues ultimately supports performance whereas a chronic inability to temporarily let go of issues results in a stunting of performance capacities. Genuine performance requires a self system that is capable of managing when issues are worked with. An unconscious compulsion to bring up issues when you need to perform almost always stunts performance and points to a necessity to develop greater personal control.

[34] Wilber, K. (1995). Sex, Ecology, Spirituality: The spirit of evolution. Boston, MA: Shambhala Publications, Inc.

The four domains are derived explicitly from Wilber's four quadrants. For an in depth look at quadrants please see Sex Ecology Spirituality.

[35] Wilber, K. Excerpt D: The Look of a Feeling: The importance of post/structuralism. Retrieved from http://wilber.shambhala.com/html/books/kosmos/excerptD/part1.cfm/

The term "inside" is being used here as how domains come to life while you are practicing Body-Mind-Moment Training. Advanced students of integral theory, please take note inside is not being used in the same context as Wilber's Integral Methodological Pluralism.

[36] Alexander, C.N., Heaton, D.P. & Chandler, H.M. (1994). Advanced Human Development in the Vedic Psychology of Maharishi Yogi: Theory and Research. In Miller, M. & Cook-Greuter, S. (Eds.), Transcendence and Mature Thought in Adulthood: The Further Reaches of Adult Development (39-70). Lanham, MD: Rowman & Littlefield.

[37] Alexander, C.N., Rainforth, M.V. & Gelderloos, P. (1991). Transcendental Meditation, Self-actualization, and Psychological Health: A Conceptual overview and statistical meta-analysis. Journal of Social Behavior and Personality, 6(5), 189-247.

[38] Harung, H. S., Heaton, D.P., Graff, W.W. & Alexander, C.N. (1996). Peak Performance and Higher States of Consciousness: A study of world-class performers. Journal of Managerial Psychology, 11(4), 2-23.

[39] Travis, F. (1979). The Transcendental Meditation Technique and Creativity: A longitudinal study of Cornell University undergraduates. Journal of Creative Behavior, 13 (3), 169-180.

[40] Flugel Colle, K.F., Vincent, A., Cha, S.S., Loehrer, L.L., Bauer, B.A. & Wahner-Roedler, D.L. (2010). Measurement of Quality of Life and Participant Experience with the Mindfulness-based Stress Reduction Program. Contemporary Therapies in Clinical Practice, 16(1), 36-40.

[41] Kember, P. (1985). The Transcendental Meditation Technique and Postgraduate Academic Performance. British Journal of Educational Psychology, 55(2), 164-166.

[42] Moore, A. & Malinowski, P. (2009). Meditation, Mindfulness and Cognitive Flexibility. Consciousness and Cognition, 18(1), 176-186.

[43] Cranson, R.W., Orme-Johnson, D.W., Gackenbach, J., Dillbeck, M.C., Jones, C.H. & Alexander, C.N. Transcendental Meditation and improved performance on intelligence-related measures: A longitudinal Study. Personality and Individual Differences, 12(10), 1105-1116.

[44] Dillbeck, M.C. (1982). Meditation and Flexibility of Visual Perception and Verbal Problem Solving. Memory & Cognition, 10(3), 207-215.

[45] Gelderloos, P. (1987). Psychological Health and Development of Students at Maharishi International University: A controlled longitudinal study. Modern Science & Vedic Science, 1(4), 471-487.

[46] Shecter, H. (1977). The Transcendental Meditation Program in the Classroom: A Psychological Evaluation. Dissertation Abstracts International, 38(7), 3372.

[47] Jonsson, C. (1975). Organizational Development Through the Transcendental Meditation Program and Certain Efficiency Criteria (Unpublished Master's Thesis). Department of Business Administration, Stockholm University, Stockholm, Sweden.

[48] Nidich, S.I. (1975). A Study of the Relationship of the Transcendental Meditation Program to Kohlberg's Stages of Moral Reasoning. Dissertation Abstracts International, 36, 4361-4362.

[49] Travis, F., Arenander, A., & DeBois, D. (2004). Psychological and Physiological Characteristics of a proposed object-referral/self-referral continuum of self-awareness. Consciousness and Cognition, 13(2), 401-420.

[50] Dillbeck, M.C., Orme-Johnson, D.W. & Wallace, R.K. (1981). Frontal EEG Coherence, H-reflex, Concept Learning, and the TM-Sidhi Program. International Journal of Neuroscience, 15(3), 151-157.

[51] So Kam-Tim (1995). Testing and Improving Intelligence and Creativity in the Chinese Culture with Maharishi's Vedic Psychology: Toward a holistic and Universal Assessment (Unpublished doctoral dissertation). Department of Psychology, Maharishi International University, Fairfield Iowa, USA.

[52] Compton, W.C. & Becker, G.M. (1983). Self-actualizations and experience with zen meditation: Is a learning period necessary for mediation? Journal of Clinical Psychology, 39(6), 925-929.

[53] Orme-Johnson, D. (1987). Medical Care Utilization and the Transcendental Meditation Program. Psychosomatic Medicine, 49(5), 43-507.

[54] Wallace, R.K., Dillbeck, M., Jacobe, E. & Harrington, B. (1982). The Effects of the Transcendental Meditation and TM-Sidhi Program on the Aging Process. International Journal of Neuroscience, 16(1), 53-58.

[55] Miller, J.J., Fletcher, K. & Dabat-Zinn, J. (1995). Three-Year Follow-up and Clinical Implications of a Mindfulness Meditation-based Stress Reduction Intervention in the Treatment of Anxiety Disorders. General Hospital Psychiatry, 17(3), 192-200.

[56] Kabat-Zinn, J., et al. (1992). Effectiveness of a Meditation-Based Stress Reduction Program in the Treatment of Anxiety Disorders. The American Journal of Psychiatry, 149, 936-943.

[57] Sephton, S.E., Salmon, P., Weissbecker, I., Ulmer, C., Floyd, A., Hoover, K. & Studts, J.L. (2007). Mindfulness Meditation Alleviates Depressive Symptoms in Women with Fibromyalgia: Results of a randomized clinical trial. Arthritis Care and Research, 57(1), 77-85.

[58] Speca, M., Carlson, L.E., Goodey, E. & Angen, M. (2000). A Randomized, Wait-List Controlled Clinical Trial: The Effect of a Mindfulness Meditation-Based Stress Reduction Program on Mood and Symptoms of Stress in Cancer Patients. Psychosomatic Medicine, 62(5), 613-622.

[59] Brookes, J.S. & Scarano, T. (1985). Transcendental Meditation in the Treatment of post-Vietnam Adjustment. Journal of Counseling and Development, 64(3), 212-215.

[60] Bloomfield, H.H. (1975). Some Observations on the Uses of the Transcendental Meditation Program in Psychiatry (Unpublished doctoral dissertation). Institute of Psychophysiological Medicine, San Diego, California, USA.

[61] Sudsuang, R., Chentanez, V. & Veiuvan, K. (1991). Effect of Buddhist Meditation on Serum Cortisol and Total Protein Levels, Blood Pressure, Pulse Rate, Lung Volume and Reaction Time. Psychology & Behavior, 50(3), 543-548.

[62] Zaichkowsky, L.D. & Kamen, R. (1978). Biofeedback and Meditation: Effects on Muscle Tension and Locus of Control. Perceptual and Motor Skills, 46(3), 955-958.

[63] Wallace, R.W. (1970). Physiological Effects of Transcendental Meditation. Science, 167(3926), 1751-1754.

[64] Travis, F. & Wallace, K.R. (1999). Autonomic and EEG Patterns During Eyes-Closed Rest and Transcendental Meditation(TM) Practice: The Basis for a Neural Model of TM Practice. Consciousness and Cognition, 8(3), 302-318.

[65] Lazar, S.W., et al. (2005). Meditation Experience is Associated with Increased Cortical Thickness. Neuroreport, 16(17), 1893-1897.

[66] Siegel, D., (2007). The Mindful Brain: Reflection and Attunement in the Cultivation of Well-Being. NY: WW Norton Company, Inc.

[67] Welwood, J. (1996). Reflection and Presence: The dialectic of self knowledge. The Journal of Transpersonal Psychology, 28(2), 107-128.
For an in depth discussion on journaling, phenomenological reflection and meditation please see Welwood's article.

[68] Cox, R.H. (2002). Sport Psychology: Concepts and Applications 5th edition. NY: McGraw-Hill.

[69] Joshi, L.N., Joshi, V.D. & Gokhale, L.V. (1992). Effects of short term 'Pranayam' practice on breathing rate and ventilatory functions of lung. Indian Journal of Physiology and Pharmacology, 36(2), 105-108.

[70] Brown, R.P. & Gerberg, P.L. (2005). Sudarshan Kriya Yogic Breathing in the Treatment of Stress, Anxiety, and Depression: Part I-Neurophysiologic Model. The Journal of Alternative and Complementary Medicine, 11(1), 189-201.

[71] Raju, P.S., Madhavi, S., Prasad, K.V., Reddy, M.E., Sahay, B.K., & Murthy, K.J. (1994). Comparison of effects of yoga and physical exercise in athletes. Indian Journal of Medical Research, 100, 81-86.

[72] Murry, B. (2007). Hydration and Physical Performance. Journal of the American College of Nutrition, 26(90005), 542-548.

[73] Shannon, J., White, E., Shattuck, A.L. & Potter, J.D. (1996). Relationship of food groups and water intake to colon cancer risk. Cancer Epidemiol Biomarkers Prevention, 5(7), 495-502.

[74] Grandjean, A.C. & Grandjean, N.R. (2007). Dehydration and Cognitive Performance. Journal of the American College of Nutrition, 26(5), 549S-554S.

[75] Czeiler, C. (2006). Sleep Deficit: The Performance Killer. Harvard Business Review, 84(10), 53-59.

[76] Leonard, G. & Murphy, M. (1995). The Life We Are Given: A long-term program for realizing the potential of body, mind, heart and soul. NY: Jeremy P. Tarcher / Putnam.

[77] Professionals who are training you in a specific modality will have prescriptive norms as to how much and when recovery is to be employed. This may vary greatly from what you are used to if you are new to the modality. As such, while training with experienced professionals it is best to follow their lead and then learn how best to integrate the optimal recovery processes within the structure of the Training Architecture being taught. Experienced professionals will also be reading you on a number of different levels and may be intentionally challenging you to disrupt your homeostasis. This experience is different than the novice who habitually engages in distracting social exchanges that interfere with optimal recovery. Please note, "novice" here is referring to the depth in which they work. Some professionals train people for decades as a novice while others can begin to train and instruct at refined levels within a few short years. Ultimately the depth of guidance provided is mediated by the depth of their own practice.

[78] Baty, J.J., Hwang H., Ding Z., Bernard J.R., Wang B., Kwon, B. & Ivy, J.L. (2007). The effect of a carbohydrate and protein supplement on resistance exercise performance, hormonal response, and muscle damage. Journal of Strength and Conditioning Research, 21(2), 321-329.

[79] Cribb P.J. & Hayes, A. (2006). Effects of supplement timing and resistance exercise on skeletal muscle hypertrophy. Medicine & Science in Sports & Exercise, 38(11), 1918-1925.

[80] Tipton, K.D., Rasmussen, B.B., Miller, S.L., Wolf, S.E., Owens-Stovall, S.K., Petrini, B.E. & Wolfe, R.R. (2001). Timing of amino acid-carbohydrate ingestion alters anabolic responses of muscle to resistance exercise. American Journal of Physiology, 281(2), 197-206.

[81] Coburn, J.W., Housh, D.J., Housh, T.J., Malek, M.H., Beck, T.W., Cramer, J.T., Johnson, G.O. & Donlin, P.E. (2006). Effects of leucine and whey protein supplementation during eight weeks of unilateral resistance training. Journal of Strength Conditioning and Resistance, 20(2), 284-291.

[82] A substantial portion of research has been conducted on pre-nutrition training where nutrients are consumed immediately prior to training. Therefore, you may consume your pre-training nutrients leading up to and including immediately prior to beginning your training.

[83] Miller, S.L., Tipton, K.D., Chinkes, D.L., Wolf, S.E. & Wolfe R.R. (2003). Independent and combined effects of amino acids and glucose after resistance exercise. Medicine & science in Sports & Exercise, 35(3), 449-455.

[84] Berardi, J.M., Price, T.B., Noreen, E.E. & Lemon, P.W. (2006). Postexercise muscle glycogen recovery enahnced with a carbohydrate-protein supplement. Medicine & Science in Sports & Exercise, 38(6), 1106-1113.

[85] Rasmussen, B.B., Tipton, K.D., Miller, S.L., Wolf S.E. & Wolfe, R.R. (2000). An oral essential amino acid-carbohydrate supplement enhances muscle protein anabolism after resistance exercise. Journal of Applied Physiology, 88(2), 386-392.

[86] During training nutrient timing is an alternative and or supplementary third option for nutritional recovery. Research has supported this practice and its effectiveness for increasing protein synthesis and decreasing protein breakdown. If you are interested in leveraging 'during training' nutrient timing into your practice of recovery, find a qualified nutritionist to tailor a strategy that supports your specific training demands.

Lightning Source UK Ltd.
Milton Keynes UK
UKOW04n2300100915

258381UK00002B/17/P